THE MAGUIRE METHOD

THE HANDBOOK FOR UNLOCKING SUCCESS AND HAPPINESS IN THE NEW AGE

CJ JOHNSON

ISBN: 979-8-8689-7673-5

Printed in the United States of America.

CONTENTS

Sunrises

The average person makes around 35,000 choices per day. Today, I chose to come to a familiar place. I'm standing on a shoreline, watching the rising sun peak over the ocean's horizon. Toes in the sand.

I always end up here. It's true what they say, you always end up where you started, but it never quite feels the same. Never. At this moment, I am alone. The sun is hazy, a soft glowing ball of orange. Although the sea is calm, its shimmering waves foretell the chaos of crashing waves soon to come.

When someone speaks of being present and embracing the world's beauty, this is what I always imagined. It's at this moment I realize I always preferred sunrises over sunsets. Let me explain. Dawn is a new day. An awakening. It's easy to catch a sunset and notice something descending into darkness.

There is something sweet about that too. However, to catch a sunrise, it takes extra dedication to rise and embrace its beauty. I let out a long extended breath. I didn't even realize I had been holding it in for so long. I do that sometimes.

Breathing is freedom in a way. To inhale is to take in all of life's problems and challenges. To exhale is to release it all, freedom. Pause to consider the importance of a breathing exercise when it comes to meditation, health, and well-being. We live in a world of busyness to the point that we need guides to help us breathe correctly.

How strange is that? Knowing how quickly a moment can pass makes me wish this moment would never end. When it passes, what will I do then? I feel guilty for letting my mind wander to what comes next instead of appreciating what's happening now. Even worse, I feel guilty for taking this moment to myself in the first place.

Especially when I have so many other things I can be doing. Why is that? To reflect on a time that came before us. That is, the notion of having a slower-paced lifestyle. How did the world function for centuries without technology as we know it today?

I wish I could just appreciate the now and not worry about a future that has yet to come. I wrote this book because I wanted to offer you a brand new perspective to help you live your best life, whatever that means for you. With a tap, a swipe, or a click, our lives have become more automated thus more convenient. That convenience is a blessing that those that came before us never got the privilege of experiencing. Even then, this convenience comes at a price with a loss of self, an overwhelming amount of distractions, an inflation of ego, increasing depression/anxiety, and an emphasis on avoidance.

This has disrupted and cluttered our everyday lives and has made it more difficult to have real connection with one another and even worse with ourselves. The truth is that the things you want the most in life will always require a tumultuous challenge. It won't be convenient and there won't be any instant gratification. The best things in life do not come easy. This book is about choices.

The choices that reshape our lives. I often felt guilty when I would enjoy the sunrises to myself just for a self-imposed time-out to recharge my own batteries. I would return to time-sensitive work emails, texts of *why r u ignoring me*? or missed calls from my family checking in on me. Then there was that itch to pick up my mobile device, check on social media with an egocentric tug to share my own opinions and insights for people that never requested it in the first place.

But I have to share, don't I? Everyone else. How else will they know I'm alive and well? We live in uncertain times and this book is for those of you who want to be seen and heard in this world. This book will help you discover (or even re-discover) how you can leave a mark in this world and live a fulfilled life.

When I was asked who this book is for I would always reply, "Well, this is for everyone." I have discovered that although each of us has our own views of the world we do have more in common that brings us together than separates us. So, read this book if the following applies to you:

- You're trying to repair a broken heart.
- You're feeling stuck in life.
- You're not sure how to find your place in the world.
- You're unsure how to navigate the evolving complex social norms.
- The world is changing and you're having trouble just dealing with it.
- You're battling anxiety and depression.
- You got what you wanted but not sure what should come next.

- Everything is going well but you want more (whatever *more* is).
- You just want to learn something new.

Most importantly, if this book caught your attention and you're reading it, this book simply put… is meant for YOU. From emerging generations that are still discovering themselves in our new world to the older generations that are grappling with a new reality. We are both one and the same, trying to make sense of the fast-changing world, and our place in it. I crafted a four-principle method to provide you with insights, resources, strategies, and tools to help you truly live the life you always imagined for yourself even with the challenges you're facing in today's world – *The Maguire Method.*

Why is it called *The Maguire Method*? The name was inspired as a tongue-in-cheek reference to one of my all-time favorite films, *Jerry Maguire.* Jerry Maguire is a successful sports agent who seemingly has everything: he's wealthy, powerful, respected, handsome, charming, has the most prominent clients, and even has a beautiful fiancée. One night, Jerry questions his purpose and place in the world. It's a story of self-discovery in a cynical world. It's true that you can find inspiration in all things.

For me, it was more than just a romcom. The film's underlying themes of examining the ego, minimalism, and prioritizing love and friendships in a world that often suggests you do otherwise was an obvious commentary about the world in which we live in. To think, the 1996 film is just as relevant today as it was back then. *The Maguire Method* is broken down into four easy-to-understand core principles. Within each core principle there will be strategies, exercises, and techniques you can apply to your life to truly achieve the life you always dreamed.

These principles are the following:

1. Questions
2. Reflections
3. Actions
4. Habits

Questions: This is the first principle of *The Maguire Method*. When we ask better questions of ourselves and the world around us, it empowers us.

Reflections: This principle allows us to come up with the answers we were asking from our first principle with clarity which informs our future mindsets and actions.

Actions: When we use our first two principles, we have a clearer path to achieving our desires, understanding our motivations, and ultimately the steps we need to take to get what we want. It only makes sense that what comes next is to take bold action. You will discover the type of action that will get you the best results you're looking for.

Habits: Our final principle is the most critical component of leveling up and ultimately transforming your life. It's taking our first three principles and taking what you have learned in this book and using it to make it a part of your lifestyle.

Each principle is intertwined with one another and you will learn how you can apply this method with increasing efficiency to your life. With the principles we will explore in this book, you will have some peace of mind to know that no matter your circumstances, there are things that you can do to empower yourself.

You can become the best version of yourself in a way you have never thought possible. As you read on, I hope that you can absorb what you feel will help you the most on your life's journey. Leave the rest. Share what you think is worth sharing. Empower yourself and empower others around you.

CHAPTER ONE

It Begins With Something New

It's essential that you know who I am. Where I come from. Every failure, tough lesson learned, and triumph led me to writing this very book to pass on what I learned to you. The most significant moment of my life began with something new. It was the birth of my first daughter, Fiona. It's true what they say, your life changes when you become a parent. Before she arrived, her mother and I went through nine months of various emotions.

There were times when we felt swallowed up by the darkness of fatigue, fear of the unknown, and anxiety. Other times, there were tidal waves of excitement at the thought of adding a new member to our family. We did typical things that would welcome the arrival of a newborn plus quirky stuff like reading to my wife's stomach and putting headphones on her belly to play music. Fiona was born in a dramatic and somewhat scary fashion. She was overdue and although we had a birth plan in place, we had to abandon it for an emergency c-section.

The entire process happened at warp speed like a smashmouth scene out of a medical drama. Our doctor was an all-around badass. A beautiful Black woman with a large yellow afro, our doctor shouted orders like a drill sergeant. She moved with precision and-Boom! Fiona was introduced to the world. They rushed her to the opposite end of our large room, in the corner.

Everyone moved quickly, attending to the baby, others taking care of my wife. As I clutched onto my wife's hand, she whispered to me in the softest tone I've ever heard, "I can't hear the baby." She was right. I couldn't either. The way she said it in her faint tone, I was scared shitless that something was very wrong. After a few tense minutes, Fiona finally let out her first cry.

The most miraculous and unforgettable moment of my life happened next. She cried so loudly that the nurses moved even faster to guide me over to her. The nurse said, "Mr. Johnson, say hello to your baby girl."

I said, "Hey Fiona." She stopped crying, turned to me with a hint of recognition, and smiled.

From that day forward, my life was never the same. Life has this funny way of never working out the way you intended. In some ways, it is even better than you could ever dream. In other ways, quite the opposite. For me, Fiona's mother, and I would end up divorcing a couple of years after she was born.

I would spend the next few years in a whirlwind of romances, business endeavors, and career shifts. All while trying to navigate being Fiona's dad and embarking on my own journey of self-discovery. During this time, I discovered my true purpose in inspiring others, and discovering *The Maguire Method*. For you to understand why I felt the need to do this in the first place. I would like to briefly take you back to the beginning. The beginning for me was when I was born on December 16th in a small town outside of Memphis, Tennessee.

I'm the son of a career U.S. Army Officer who was raised in

the south by my great-grandmother, lovingly called "Big Mama." He witnessed first-hand the intensity of the civil rights movement. My grandmother herself often told me stories of her activism, marching through the streets. From what I know, her first husband also served in the U.S. military. She and her second husband, a car mechanic (whom I consider being my great grandfather, "Papa"), were entrepreneurial caretakers of their local neighborhood.

Later in life, Big Mama got Alzheimer's and lived with my family until her eventual passing. Around the same time, my Papa mysteriously wound up in Los Angeles at Cedar Sinai. How? It still remains a mystery. Days before he died, I was informed by a "cousin" I had never met before where he was.

When I last saw him, he was in a comatose state, shriveled up, on his last days. Once, a strong man whose fingers were so large he bruised my ribs when he tickled me faded away in front of me. My father was a very complicated man of mystery to me as well. He was the strong but silent type and a charismatic leader. My mother was a firecracker, constantly pushing my younger sister and me to great lengths.

While in college, she became pregnant with me and dropped out of school. But as a child, I saw her go back to school to complete achieving her degree with me in tow. My parents were two people that came from difficult childhoods and dedicated their lives to perseverance and excellence. Although they were both strict disciplinarians, they allowed me and my younger sister to freely express ourselves. I suppose they didn't have much of a choice.

I spent most of my life moving from place to place because of my father's military career. Just a few months after I was born, my family moved to Germany, where I learned to speak German before I learned English. I had a nanny named Bergata. Her husband and teenage punk rock daughter, Sasha, treated me like a family member. I can't remember their faces, but I still remember the loving embrace they gave me.

From there, we never lived anywhere longer than four years. I got accustomed to various labels from "new kid" to "class clown". I understood majestic beginnings and bittersweet endings far sooner than most. I also had to learn how to adapt to new environments quickly, always having to embrace different people of different cultures. At 17, my family moved to the Marshall Islands during the summer of my senior year of high school.

The island, a U.S. missile testing site, is three miles long and one mile wide. On this island, a blonde hippie woman taught me not just how to swim but also the unforgettable lesson of going with the flow instead of fighting against the current. I remember the rhythm in which she spoke to me, teaching me how to swim. She offered me sage wisdom through the art of learning how to swim. Up until this point, I was just trucking along, avoiding swimming at all costs.

I was terrified of water. I had multiple experiences of my dad trying to teach me how to swim at an early age by throwing me in the pool and dunking my head under water, hoping I would just figure it out. I didn't. Then there was the time an older cousin pushed me in the deep end of a tide pool and a lifeguard had to save me from drowning. To add to my phobia of water was that I watched countless movies about predators lurking in the depths of the ocean with a taste for human blood to tales of being lost at sea. Yet there I was learning how to swim for the first time in the Pacific Ocean.

I learned first-hand from even that one experience that there is a clear difference between going with the flow and just trucking along. Going with the flow is about having a deeper understanding of yourself, the world around you. You can use a combination of chaos and order to create your own destiny the way you see fit and accept fate as it is. The latter is like being a pawn in a chess game with or without your willing participation.

That wouldn't be the only lesson learned. There were many more to come. That would happen a lot in my life. I was more drawn to adults than to peers my own age. From playing my first Nintendo video game with the three ROTC dudes who lived down the street to purposefully get detention so I could stay after school to help my crush, the art teacher, tidy up her classroom.

I remember the first time I was heartbroken at 17, getting love advice from a drunken first sergeant over a glass of Irish whiskey. That was pretty normal for me. I was always guided, mentored, and supported by men and women from various backgrounds. They all had one thing in common. They were open about sharing their life experiences and passing down lessons they learned. Each person was amused by my eagerness to learn something new. Each of them kindly took the time to offer me words of advice.

For example, my Godparents, a doctor and a former police officer turned entrepreneur, stressed the importance of being an outspoken member of the community and empowering the voiceless. I was never fond of social constructs or doing what was the status quo. If I wasn't interested in conventionally doing things. For example, when I was 13 years old, my father demanded that I add cutting our lawn to my list of chores. The first day I was supposed to start doing this, he arrived home to find my best friend mowing our front yard.

He found me on the front porch peacefully reading a comic

book when he approached our house. He asked what the hell was going on. I informed him that I took a portion out of my allowance to hire my friend to cut our lawn. When my father responded, I can't for the life of me remember what he angrily grumbled. Because at that very moment, I came up with the idea to go to each house in the neighborhood and offer my friend's services to cut their lawn.

For a small fee, of course. If I wasn't interested in typical social norms, I especially wasn't interested in the way the world around me tried to force racial stereotypes on me. I refused to let anyone rob my happiness, innocence, freedom, and success. In fact, I spent my life challenging stereotypes and limiting beliefs about what a Black person should or shouldn't be. The thing about any biases and stereotypes is that people throw their beliefs, values, and perspectives onto you without any intention of actually getting to know you as you truly are.

Bizarrely, if you challenge their limiting beliefs, you are an anomaly. An exception to made-up rules that were built by *they*. Whoever the fuck *they* is, it never mattered to me. There are always lessons to be learned in competitive sports, especially ones where you are matched up in one-on-one duels. This led to me being a very scrappy kid growing up. As a globetrotting Black kid, I got to hear different iterations of the n-word, and in return, I learned how to pack a punch. In fact, this made me more drawn to martial arts, wrestling, and boxing.

I learned a particular lesson early on at the age of 9. I took karate, and in a sparring match, I fought a kid who matched me blow for blow. Then out of nowhere, he punched me in my stomach. It was the first time I ever got the air knocked out of me. I was pretty dramatic about it.

I dropped to my knees, doubled over, gasping for air. On the silent drive home, my embarrassment only grew. I cried so hard everyone just watched, stunned for a moment. My biggest disappointment was looking over to see my dad watching. When we got home, he asked me how I felt. I told him how embarrassed and caught off guard I was.

He replied softly that we would make sure that wouldn't happen again. For the next week, my father would randomly punch me in the stomach with sneak attacks. Other times he practiced karate moves with me. Alone, I'd hit my stomach repeatedly to toughen up. When I finally faced off with this kid again for a rematch, I was ready for whatever he would throw at me. Exactly like last time we traded blows.

Evenly matched until he went for the same move he did last time. I didn't bother blocking it. I just absorbed the punch. He was stunned that I had no reaction and quickly punched me in the stomach again. Within a split second, I side-kicked as hard as I could in his stomach.

This time he was the one on the floor crying. This lesson taught me whatever life throws at you, it's up to you how you react to it. It's up to you how you respond. Each of us has our own journey. We all react to the world around us differently.

Every successful and happy person has a different playbook and individual sense of self that helps propel them to what they achieve. The common starting point always starts with you. You can shape your world into the way you want for yourself. For you to do that, you must embrace a growth mindset. Embracing a growth mindset separates those who "get it" and those who "don't."

In a growth mindset, people believe their most basic abilities can be developed through dedication and hard work. Brains and talent are just the starting point. This perspective creates a love of learning and resilience that is essential for significant accomplishments. I decided to take all of the lessons I learned throughout life and go forward with a growth mindset. Even as I navigated This played a critical role in the success and experience that followed.

I would eventually become an award-winning Photographer, Filmmaker, and even Marketer. I have successfully contributed to hundreds of startups and Fortune 500 companies of various industries. I would become one of the leading global minds on the creator economy, brand strategy, social media marketing, and cultural consumer trends. Advisory board roles for non-profits, startup accelerators, and small businesses would soon follow. As life's journey presented windy roads that led to places I never imagined I continued on with this growth mindset.

I even found a way to share my journey through creative storytelling and lifestyle tips amassing hundreds of thousands of social media followers. I became known as a "dot connector", recognizing trends and patterns early to help others understand how these shifts impact culture and consumer behavior in all industries. This led to me being featured in publications like *GQ Magazine*, *Forbes*, *Men's Health*, *Huffington Post*, *Fox News*, and more. However, none of the success made me impervious to growing pains. Growing pains that were exacerbated by the rapidly changing world around me because of social identities, issues, politics, technology.

I wondered aloud and privately if I was the only one experiencing this. So, I used the power of social media as an outlet to creatively express myself and my thoughts. I hyper-focused on lifting people up and would routinely offer words of encouragement, even blocking out times out of my day just for complete strangers to video chat with me if they needed someone to just... listen. My social presence and following grew even more when I would ask more thought-provoking questions publicly that provided me more insight into how people were feeling.

Questions like, "Which would you rather have money or love?", "Would you rather rekindle a romance or a friendship?", etc. This offered a brand new perspective of what mattered the most to people. In my career, most of the roles I served as, I was considered a third party entity, always looking into a system that was either established or in the beginning stages of development. My role is always to see what's working, what's not, and how what's not working can be improved. This led to various problem-solving techniques and discovering the true motivations of decision-making.

This all played a role in how I first developed *The Maguire Method* and why I felt so inclined to create in the first place. I always found that there is synergy between our work, growth, and relationships that often gets overlooked. Especially when someone says they're trying to have better work-life balance which is essentially saying that they are feeling overwhelmed by one aspect of their life versus another. This can be exacerbated if you have a scarce mindset.

The main issue with a scarcity mindset is that it's much easier to have, especially in the modern world we live in. Having a scarce mindset means you are so obsessed with a lack of something (usually time, love, or money) that you can't seem to focus on anything else. It doesn't matter how hard you try. It turns you into the person that sees life as a finite pie.

So, if someone takes a big piece, that leaves less for everyone else. Especially you. Most of us have been conditioned to think that's true, thus having a scarcity mentality. What makes this mentality even tougher for us to break free from are the distractions that we face every single day and the reinforcement of our limiting beliefs. A limiting belief is a story we tell ourselves that we're not good enough and that we don't deserve the type of happiness we truly desire.

This ultimately leads to limiting behaviors. We need to break free of all limitations to give us the confidence to find our purpose. Humans have this deep need for stability and predictability (even if it works against us). Routines help us conserve mental energy and stay in our comfort zones to keep us from feeling anxious and getting hurt (emotionally and physically). This also keeps us in unfulfilling jobs and unhealthy relationships.

With *The Maguire Method* we are going to break free from scarcity. Continue reading with an open mind and a growth mindset. Be ready to look within and apply what you learned in your everyday life. This will allow you to absorb key information from our core principles and create more opportunities to use to your fullest advantage.

PRINCIPLE I

QUESTIONS

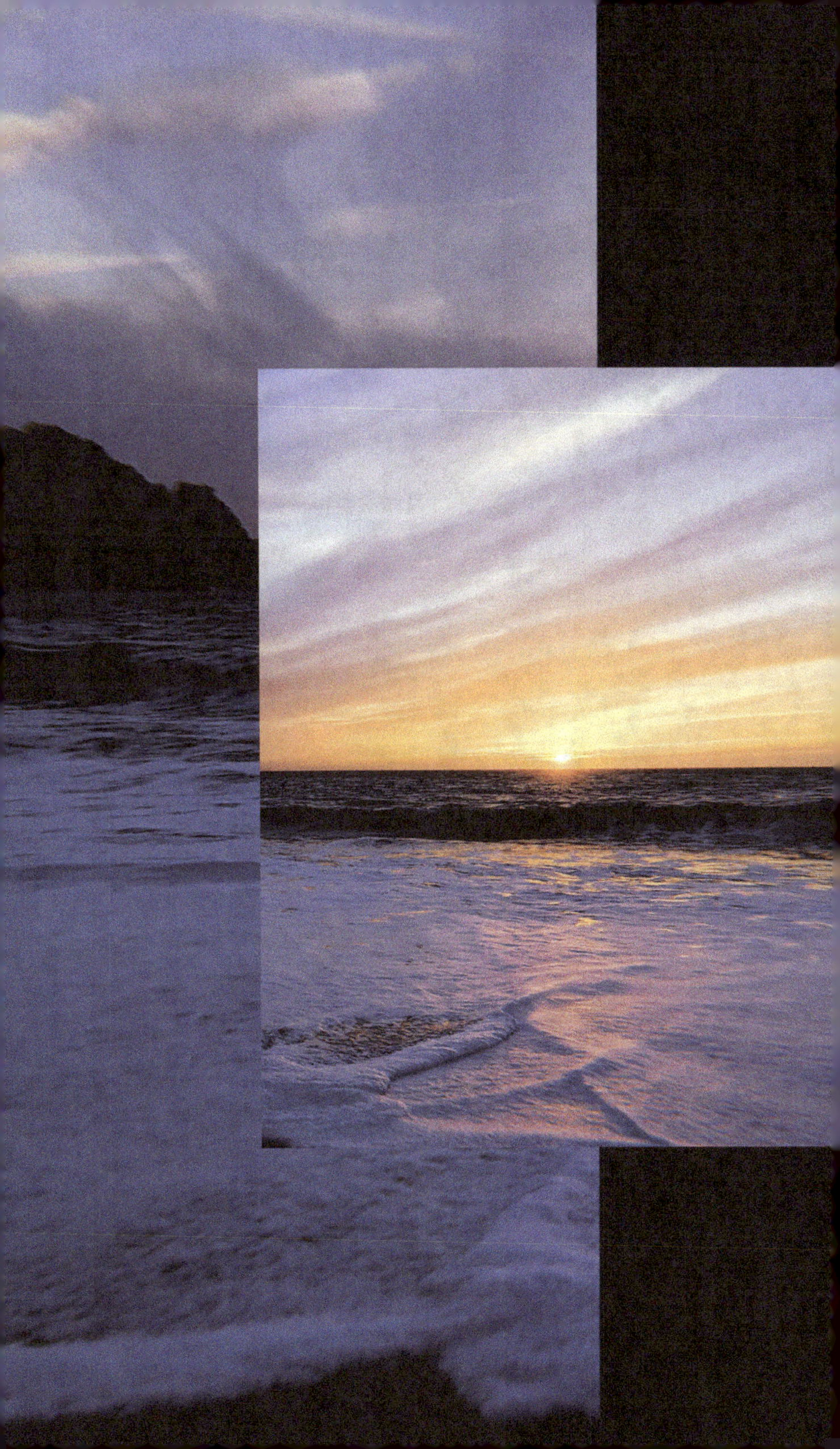

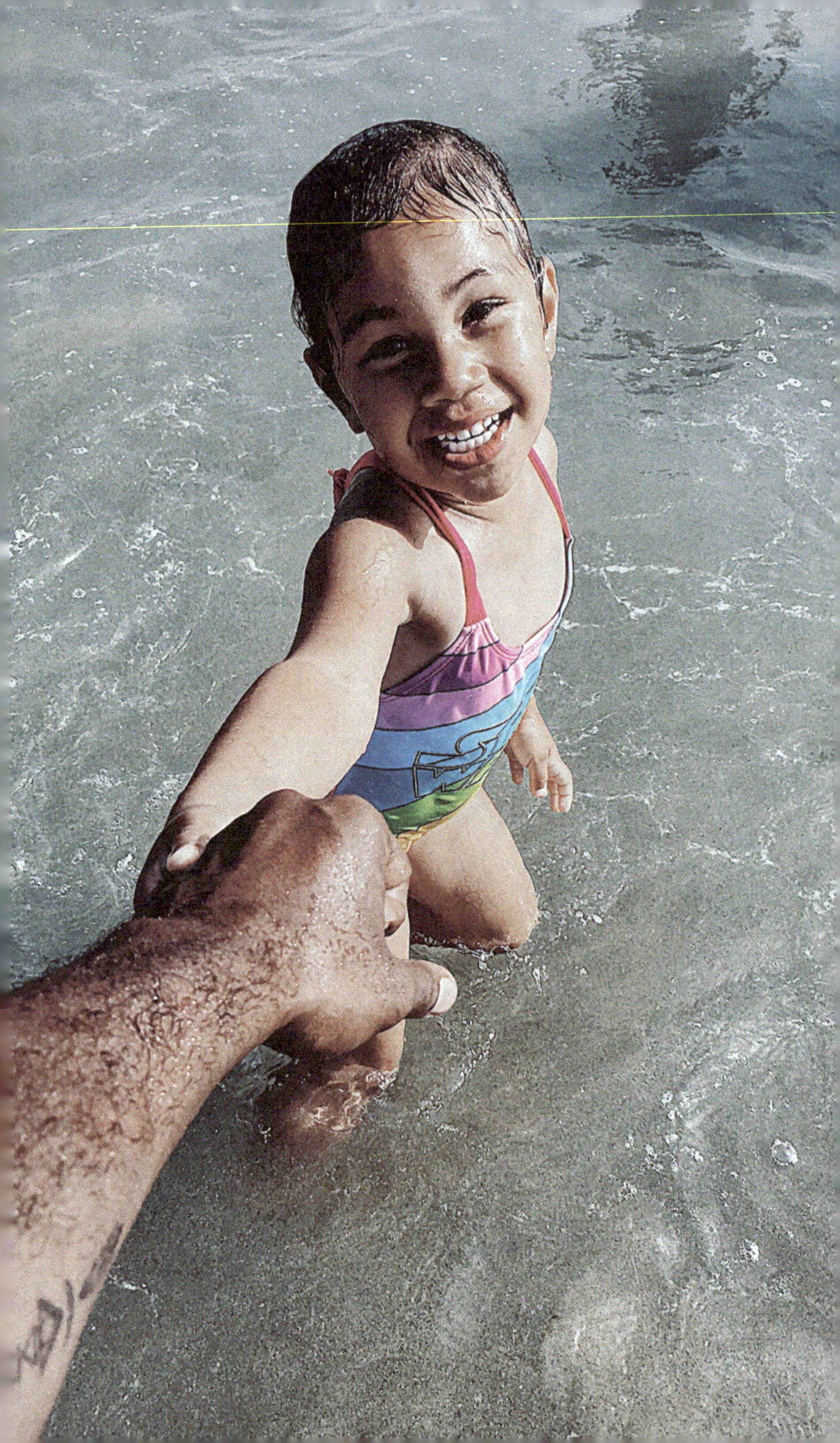

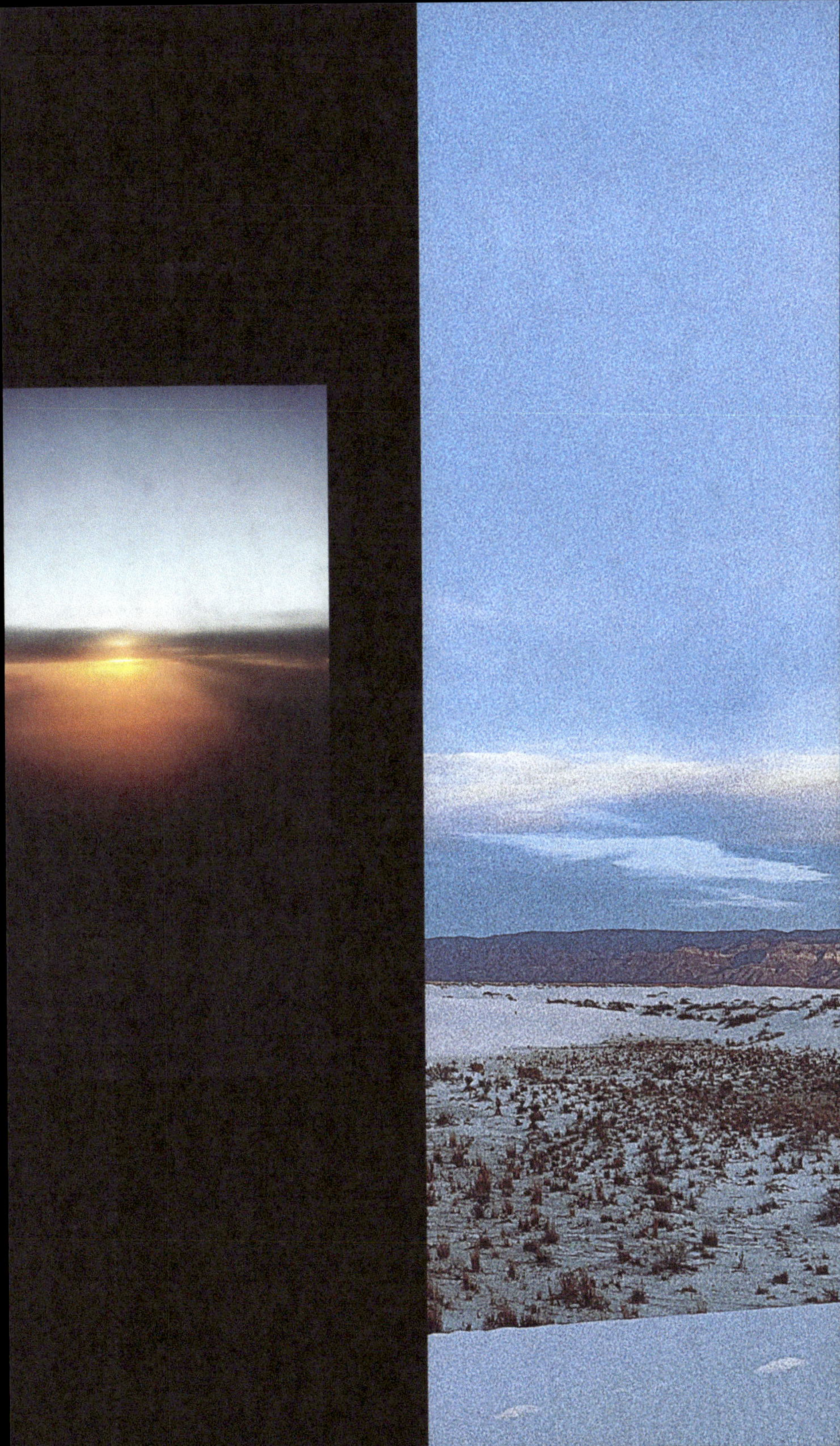

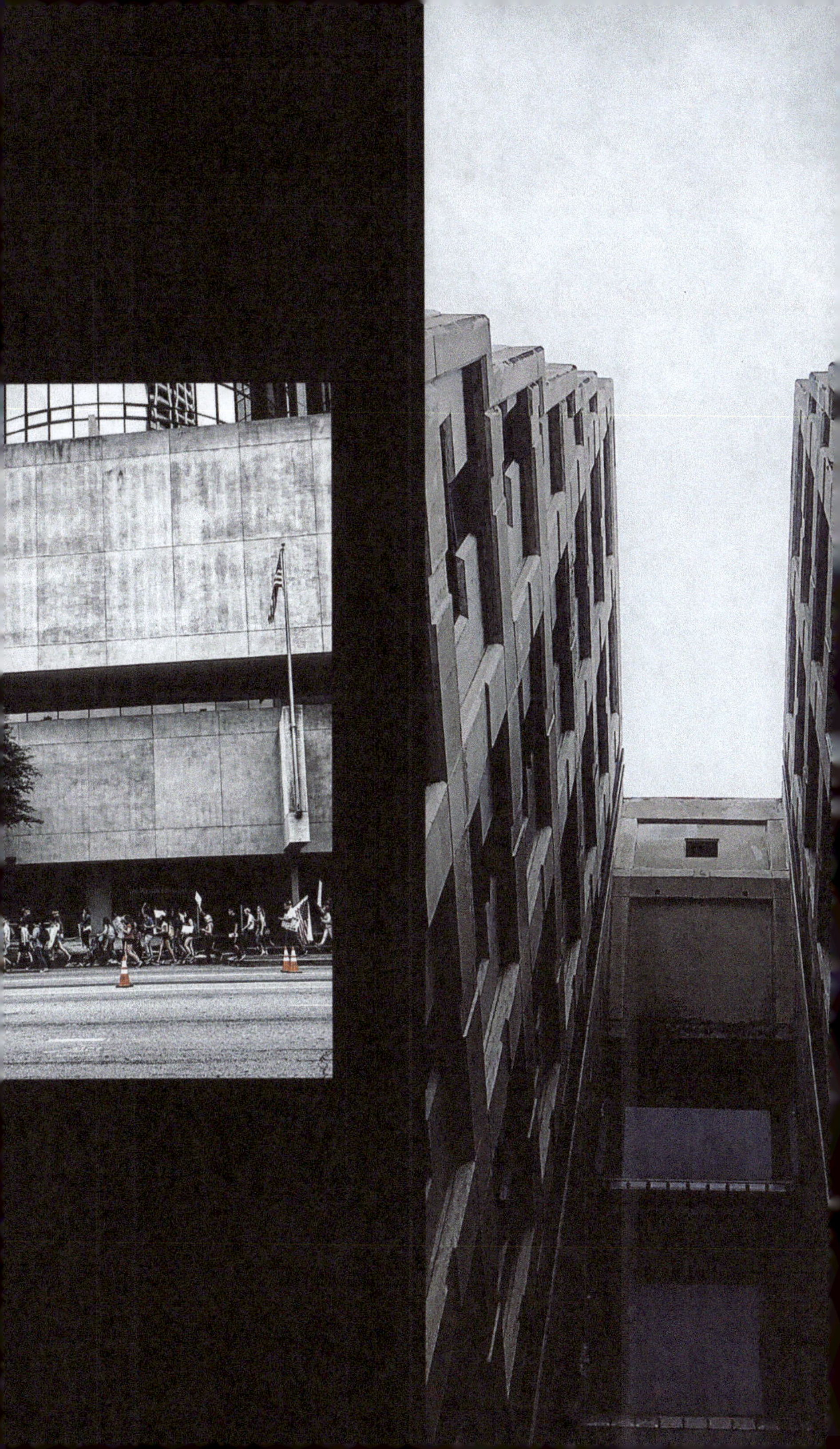

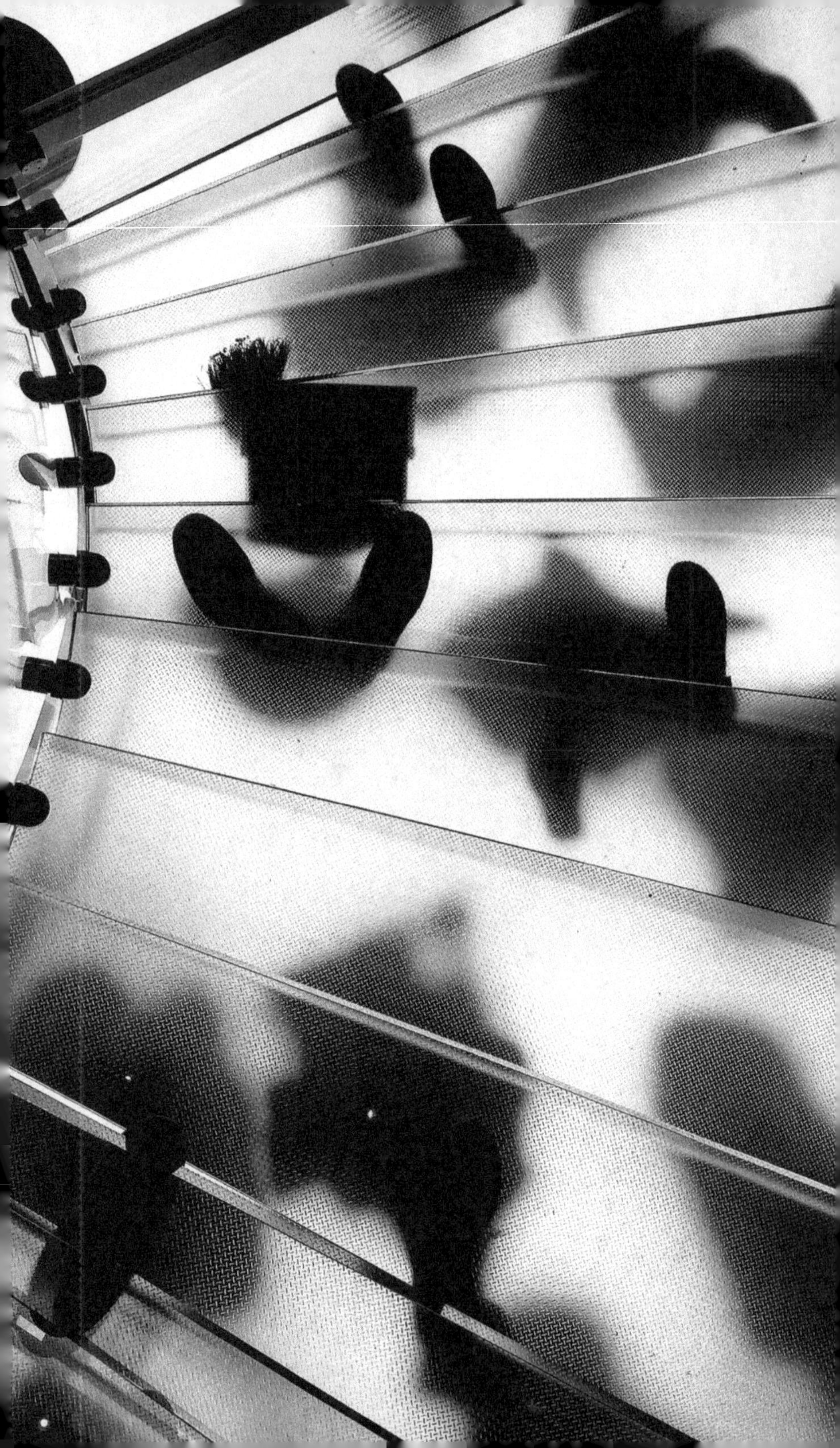

CHAPTER TWO

What Are You About... Really?

Ask questions. This is the first principle of *The Maguire Method*. It's also the best starting point for us to truly discover how you can empower yourself. When you ask questions, it will lead you down a path of self-awareness and stability that can reshape your entire universe. Asking a question sounds simple enough. Ask a question, get an answer. In a practical way, questions mitigate fears and destroy abstract challenges our minds conjure up.

It puts you into a state of mind where you're problem-solving. You may not find all of the answers you're looking for, but more often than not, if you ask the right ones, you will. We often spend more time asking the wrong questions than the right ones. I have discovered that nearly all conflicts come from a form of miscommunication within yourself and the world around you. Thus, we must actively practice more thoughtfulness to habitually ask the right questions.

When we do this, we gain clarity, perspective, knowledge, and peace of mind. This ultimately levels us up inwardly and outwardly. Depending on the framing of your questions, you can ask good ones and bad ones. We want you to ask the good ones.

By practicing this habit, you're stretching and rewiring your brain to activate differently.

Strengthening those muscles through repetition will make this process more rewarding than not. Examples of the bad questions are, "If I take a risk to follow my own dreams, I wonder what people would think of me if I fail?" or "Why doesn't this person like me?" An example of a good question would be, "Has worrying about what others think of me helped me or held me back?" The first two questions bring about self-doubt and negatively challenge your sense of self-worth. They're the wrong questions to ask.

The latter question challenges you to be thoughtful and put things into perspective. Then it nudges you to be practical about what is true. This is a good question because no matter the answer you provide, you're taking a step toward growth (inwardly and outwardly). It also allows you the opportunity to be honest about your own values and beliefs.

Before we explore the types of questions you should and shouldn't be asking, you first need to be clear on your core values and beliefs. Once you're clear on both this will provide you more clarity on how you can be more intentional with your decision making thus getting more of the results you're looking for that will make a bigger impact for yourself and others. You can discover this by asking yourself, "Do I know my own values and core beliefs? What are they?" Your belief system is a collection of the most deeply held, fundamental beliefs you hold about yourself. They can exist consciously or subconsciously.

Our beliefs substantially shape our perceptions, thoughts, emotions, and actions. We typically accept these beliefs as accurate because they are based on our accrued experiences. This last part is critical because this is how biased beliefs and perspectives can lurk in our subconscious. You see, your beliefs are also the thoughts you repeatedly think about. Your subconscious mind takes them over and starts to take hold of them as the absolute truth.

When this happens, you are no longer aware of your core beliefs. You simply think, that's *just the way I am.*

Here are a few examples of beliefs:

- Everyone is doing the best they can.
- My failure is a learning tool.
- I can do anything, but I can't do everything.
- Minor improvements are enough.
- Good things often take time.

When you understand more about your beliefs, you're able to use this as a cheat code to discover who you are and what you're all about. This leads to your core values. Your core values are traits or qualities that represent your highest priorities, deeply held beliefs, and fundamental driving forces. When it comes to understanding our values, everyone is entirely different.

Let's try this exercise of asking good questions to learn more about what your values are:

Who do you admire? An easy way to better understand what you value is to simply turn to real-life examples of your positive role models or people who have admirable qualities that inspire you. This includes people you know personally, famous figures, characters in your favorite movie, etc. What about them inspires you? What type of behaviors do they have that you would like to emulate?

What inspires you to take action? Our core values reveal themselves through our own actions. Think about the times you took bold action for yourself or others. What motivated you to take action? Think about what you gained or lost when you took it. What were you willing to risk in that situation?

When do you feel most like yourself? You should walk in integrity with yourself. You do that, win or lose. You're living on your own terms. When you're in situations that allow you to be authentic, that's a critical clue that you align with your values. For example, have you ever been in a situation where you felt that you betrayed yourself in order to fit in or find success? Did you feel ashamed and alone? In case something feels wrong in some way, explore what's going on.

When you're feeling ashamed, alone, or not in alignment, ask yourself:

- Who were you with?
- What feelings were triggered?
- What did those experiences cost you emotionally or physically?

When you're feeling authentic, what does it feel like to be in alignment with yourself?

- Who were you with?

- What activities were involved?
- Where were the positive emotions or outcomes of these experiences?

When you can answer those questions, you're empowering yourself and others around you. Once you have those answers for yourself, you can simplify things a bit to explore which values mean the most to you. Here are some examples of core values to get you started:

- Family
- Freedom
- Security
- Loyalty
- Sportsmanship
- Responsibility
- Respect
- Integrity
- Creativity

Now, if you were to apply your values to your belief system, it might look something like this:

- Integrity - I know and do what is right.
- Respect - I will treat others the way I want to be treated.
- Responsibility - I will embrace opportunities to contribute.

Understanding your own core values and beliefs is like having a special type of armor that protects you from the slings and arrows that the world sends at you. There has never come a more critical time to understand more about yourself than now. We live in a world where everything from facts to reality to even our sense of well-being is challenged every second of every day. If you're not careful, getting lost in a sea of confusion is easy.

Take, for example, the growing emphasis and importance of our digital lives, which are just as (if not in some cases more) important than our in-person lives. Think about the presence of social media and its critical role in your everyday life. One can't help but think about how large of an influence it has on how we see each other and how we impact the world around us. After all, social media is where you get to share your opinions and your life with everyone else. If each and every one of us wants a sense of belonging before we perish, a social media presence is easy validation for that.

This is both good and bad. It's great because the original intent of social media leans more into the social part. You have access to various cultures and societies worldwide. You can reconnect with old friends, find a lost love, or stay in touch with your family with ease. You can even have access to celebrities, politicians, and brands you wouldn't usually have access to. All around the world!

The bad part of this is how a digital lifestyle demands so much of your attention and brain power. It also drains you of your emotional, mental, and, yes, even physical energy because you're constantly reacting to things versus being proactive. It can even inflate your ego and, without you consciously being aware, give away your sense of self-importance to the hands of online users. In so many cases, you can even turn your own social media presence into a lucrative career.

This can shape our mindsets in such a way that your opinion

and the opinions of others can easily become facts in your mind. This provides no room for growth and warps our sense of well-being. We knowingly and unknowingly attribute our intrinsic value to a *like*. This is further backed up by studies from researchers at the University of Texas at Austin who employed an experimental social media task over three studies. The team found that teenagers who received fewer *likes* during a standardized social media interaction felt more strongly rejected, and reported more negative thoughts about themselves.

Behind the scenes, the gamification of social media ensured by endorphins was created to keep us hooked. Social media companies designed their apps to stimulate parts of our brain to keep us using services that profit off of our emotional ties to it. After all, a social media feed acts like a slot machine. You scroll through your social feed with anticipation that you might land on something that you find interesting. That's the reward.

There is even a bit of excitement that comes when you scroll so much that the feed has to load to give you more options. Sometimes you lose. That's when you don't see anything you find interesting. Sometimes you win. When something catches your eye. You send a *like* as a reward.

What is more common is that some social media users go straight to the comments section of a social post just to respond to the comments. If we agree with a comment, then that user gets our approval. If not, they will feel our wrath. There is something to be said that social media has evolved and will continue to over time by changing its algorithm to keep you even more hooked based on your own habits using the platforms. This has allowed social media to show you more of what the algorithms think you want to see, offering you less of what you don't, so you are a happy camper staying put… continuing to use the slot machine.

The reward you receive is a dopamine release. When you get a social media notification, your brain sends you a reward pathway, making you feel good. Dopamine is associated with food, exercise, love, sex, gambling, drugs… and now, of course, social media. This dopamine-triggering behavior becomes habitual. Anxiety and depression are at an all-time high.

This has reshaped our society in a way in which we are becoming more addicted to feeding our egos. Just like any addictive substance, there are consequences if not done in moderation. There is no doubt that social media plays a role in this. Anxiety can destroy your body and your mind at the same time without breaking a sweat. I've seen some of the most secure people I know become completely devastated because someone else has more social media followers than they do.

Some have even obsessed about it to the point of paying for services to buy more followers and likes. Many think a higher following means what they have to say is more valid. This can make you think someone's perspective on something is more important than your own. That's not the case at all. Your perspective matters. Your voice matters.

In many ways, you may provide inspiration to someone else who needs to share their own voice. Even more remarkable is that you may be able to amplify each other and give a loud voice to the voiceless. That is good. Even when you're online and oversharing, you might want to ask yourself why you are doing it in the first place.

Ask yourself good questions to ponder how you feel about being on social media in general: "Does being on social media affect my mood? If so, how does it make me feel? Does it bother me at all? How much time do I spend on it? What kind of information do I soak in?"

The key here is to remember that we're asking more questions to clarify if we are in integrity with who we are and the world around us. If you think social media is just a way for you to express yourself and simply connect with your family and friends, I get it. You may think that "social media isn't real" and "I'm not affected by it". In reality, you actually are. Even if you're offline, there are billions of people around the world that are.

It's where most people get influential news, education, and access to family and friends. So, yes, it's okay to have a love and hate relationship with social media. Get offline if you feel that it's too much for you and affects your mood. Be mindful of why you're doing what you're doing. Simply put, keep things in perspective by being mindful of your core values when you're using social media.

CHAPTER THREE

Are You Thinking Clearly?

The truth is, we live in a world filled with distractions and an increasing comfort of confining ourselves to our own bubbles. In order for us to reclaim our own sense of purpose and clarity, we have to continue to ask ourselves better questions. Suppose you're ever on the fence about anything and seeking to gain clarity. In that case, two great questions to ask are, "Have you ever been in a situation where you weren't entirely clear if it's wishful thinking or your intuition talking" and "Am I seeing things clearly enough to make sense of things?" There is nothing more potent to our well-being than clarity. With clarity comes acceptance. What is soon to follow is peace of mind.

There are fundamental truths of human nature that you must understand when dealing with the world around us. One, not everyone sees the world the same way you do. So, in order for you to understand where someone is coming from, it's a smart move to simply ask vs. assume. This goes both ways. Not everyone is going to understand your motivations and where you come from.

We all learn the answers to this by simply getting to know one another. In a lot of cases, the truth can be confusing and even harmful if we learn someone doesn't see the world the same way we do. This is a clear example of how our ego works. If the way we perceive things isn't always right, then it directly challenges whatever narrative we have established about ourselves and the world around us. In extreme circumstances, this might feel like your voice doesn't matter, even though it really does.

Believing it doesn't is simply a self-limiting belief. Growing up, traveling around the world, and experiencing so many different cultures and lifestyles first hand I'm here to tell you everyone faces adversity and everyone has a different perspective on how they view life. We find commonality with each other by wanting to be seen and heard which ultimately boils down to each of us wanting our lives to feel significant in some way. Many people see themselves as the hero.

If you know anything about heroes or even a hero's journey, heroes like the rest of us are often flawed. Not perfect. Not impervious to the world around them. We are all human, after all. If you can be open-minded and admit if you're wrong versus trying to massage your ego and have a confirmation bias about things, you can gain clarity on any circumstance faster. Admitting you are wrong shows you are willing to grow and learn from past mistakes. If someone doubles down and shifts the blame, it makes them seem like they are stubborn.

Humans do have a tough time admitting fault. No matter who you are, it takes some courage to shatter your ego and admit your mistakes. If you're having issues realizing when you're wrong or dealing with someone else who is pushing their beliefs on you that you clearly disagree with, here are some great questions to ask yourself:

- What part of my past is this person triggering?
- Where does this send me on an emotional level?
- What types of stories am I telling myself about this person/situation?
- Do I feel reactive about this? If so, in what way?
- What do I want to do?
- Who or what does this person or situation remind me of?
- In what ways do I act like this person?
- Is there any area in my life where I also show up in this way?
- In what ways do I not act like this person? Why is that?
- Am I afraid that I might be like this person or that others might think of me in this way? If yes, what's at the core of this fear?
- What do I need to do to take care of myself right now?
- How can I self-soothe?
- How can I be compassionate while also setting a healthy boundary?

Now, that might seem like a list of complicated questions to ask yourself but remember that taking one step at a time, asking even one of the above questions, will help you get the results you need to grow faster.

Two, we need different perspectives, especially those we disagree with. Without various views on anything in life, we would have fewer opportunities for growth, change, and self-empowerment. Choose to have direct conversations with people instead of just projecting your views or, worse, avoid challenging discussions entirely. Practice empathy and tolerance. Tolerant individuals are not threatened by differing opinions or lifestyles.

In fact, they tend to be less competitive with others and do not seek to change other people's views or perspectives. Why? They focus on acceptance rather than the competition. This enables greater intimacy and makes relationships of all kinds more satisfying and healthier.

You can practice tolerance by simply honoring the opinions of others that are different from your own. This can be done through acceptance, interest, and accommodation. Here is an example of what I mean:

Neal: *Hey Dana, can you work for me this Friday night?*

Dana: *I can't. I volunteer at my church on Friday nights.*

Neal: *I didn't know that you were religious.*

Dana: *I guess so. It's just something I've done my whole life.*

Neal: *I've never been much of a religious person. I'm not sure what I believe in, but I always found religions to be a bit patriarchal. Don't you think some of the practices are outdated?*

Dana: *I can't speak for anyone else, but from my own experiences, I've had a great sense of community, love, and acceptance at my church. You're more than welcome to tag along one of these times to see how you like it. It's a lot of fun, and I am a proud member of my church. Would you be open to that?*

Neal: *It's not really my thing, but it sounds like you're enjoying it. Why don't we just arrange our schedules so that I work every Friday night, and you can work Saturday nights? Would that work better for you?*

Dana: *That would be great! Thank you.*

In the above exchange, Dana and Neal are obviously coming from two different perspectives. Neal starts by asking if Dana is available to work for him. Her response simply explains why she isn't available. But Neal decides to swerve off-topic to both ask and challenge Dana's perspective. This type of situation happens often. But Dana's response is respectful, accepting of Neal's beliefs, and then directly asks him if he's open to exploring her perspective. He's not, but he's respectful about it. They circle back to the original task and find a reasonable resolution.

Now, I'm sure you are pondering a circumstance in which you've been in a similar or even more extreme case. So, what does it look like when we practice Intolerance? Perhaps a simple topic or disagreement gets inflamed. Or maybe it's a very volatile or toxic circumstance. How do we deal with that? The anger that some individuals experience when others disagree with them is caused by the pain they feel about differing opinions or lifestyles. This is demonstrated in the following conversation between Julio and Rex right after they saw a movie together:

> Julio: *That was one of the best movies I have ever seen. It was smart, moved so fast. Wow. Can't believe how good it was. Especially that one part where-*
>
> Rex: *Really?! I could barely stand to sit through it!*
>
> Julio: *What? You didn't like it?*
>
> Rex: *Honestly, bro. The acting was shit. The story didn't make any sense at all. It was super slow. I was bored out of my mind.*
>
> Julio: *Okay. You don't know what you are talking about.*

> *Rex:*   *C'mon, man, only someone that likes dumb popcorn movies would be into that movie. Worst movie I've seen in a while to keep it real. Awful.*
>
> *Julio:*   *Wait a second. Are you calling me "dumb"?*
>
> *Rex:*   *No, I didn't say that. I said that movie was dumb.*
>
> *Julio:*   *That's not what you said. But, okay. I mean, next time, I'll go to the movies myself.*

In the above example, Julio took it personally that Rex did not like the movie that he liked and pushed Rex away because of it. Julio acted like it was his movie and became defensive of Rex's candid expression of his opinion. Why does Julio feel this way? Julio is threatened by Rex's differing opinion of the movie because he finds it invalidating. When people feel invalidated, they feel like they are crazy, stupid, or wrong for their beliefs. This is taken as a direct insult. Then they get angry, and more often than not, they lash out.

In both cases, you'll notice that the questions they were asking were argumentative versus thoughtful. There was no empathy or respect between the two. There wasn't even an opportunity to agree to disagree or even clear examples of why each one shared the opinion they did. If they did the latter, they most likely would have had a good time debating bantering about the film. The exchange, however, was just plain argumentative and toxic.

Intolerance over someone's sexual orientation is an extreme example in which some straight individuals feel so threatened by a different lifestyle that they feel the need to attack the lifestyle and those who participate. Intolerant individuals, like Julio, depend on others to validate them by agreeing with them and behaving as they do. They require that others mirror them in order to be okay with themselves in order to get along. This is a very unhealthy state and is toxic for individuals as well as society as a whole.

Tolerant individuals are self-validating. When you practice tolerance, you trust yourself to know when you are making good decisions and behave consistently in a manner that you are proud of. There isn't any reason to boost your sense of self-worth or value. Why? Because you are more secure with yourself than intolerant individuals. You are more secure because you are very clear about your values, beliefs, and boundaries. Not all is lost if you or someone you know is intolerant. In fact, you can become tolerant by learning how to self-validate rather than being dependent on others to tell you that you are not crazy, stupid, or wrong. How does one achieve the ability to self-validate?

Try these three steps:

1. Thorough self-examination and reflection (we will learn straightforward ways you can do this in our second principle). You must be willing to look at yourself critically at all times. This will allow you to be more confident in knowing yourself better than anyone else.
2. Be brutally honest with yourself. In order to validate yourself, you must trust yourself above all others. To achieve this level of trust and confidence, you must always practice asking better questions to help you be honest with yourself.
3. Consistency. Your behavior must consistently reflect your personal moral and ethical principles. This will allow you to have a more substantial capacity for tolerance. The

greater the consistency, the greater immunity you will have to the opinions of others.

Three, there is a difference between fact and opinion. Those lines are becoming increasingly blurred with misinformation. Even worse, the sources of misinformation pretend to be newsworthy facts and are often difficult to track down to the original source. But there is a line we must draw in the sand with those who spout misinformation as the truth. From conspiracy theories to misinformation to hijacking movements for political (and financial gains), we have to be more thoughtful about recognizing the lies and embracing the truth.

This is why it's so critical that we ask more questions and be clear about our own values. If we don't, this leads to polarization of views, toxicity, and even physical threats to our own lives. Clear examples of this are polarizing topics that invaded our way of life like "All Lives Matter" versus "Black Lives Matter", Cancel Culture, and Covid-19. This is why we must ask better questions. We must seek knowledge about who we are and discover how that ties into the world around us. Doing this gives you a grounded perspective on the fast-changing world around you.

It's not as easy as me listing off fact-checking websites or telling you where you need to go to see who's lying and who's telling the truth. But I can ask that you ask yourself better questions and pause before you potentially embrace ideologies based on hearsay and a tantalizing headline. It might help if you ask the following questions and see what you come up with in your answers:

Questions to ask:

- Who financially benefits from disseminating misinformation?
- Who are the producers of misinformation and disinformation?
- Where did it come from?
- Why don't people get information before they share it?
- How do I break free of my filter bubbles and echo chambers?

Remember to ask not just questions of ourselves but the world around us. We should also embrace effective communication. By prioritizing effective communication, you can increase engagement and productivity and thus boost satisfaction. The ability to communicate effectively plays a large role in avoiding confusion, resolving conflicts and preventing any potential ones from arising. Effectively communication also helps people feel more confident and understanding of expectations. The key is to make sure all parties are heard and find a solution that is ideal for everyone involved. Listening plays a pivotal role in this. If you offer a high-quality response, it helps others feel heard and understood.

Whether we're avoiding topics altogether (and even people with differing views) due to fear or discomfort about a particular topic or we're doing the opposite, embracing heated exchanges in hopes of persuading someone else to see things our way or deflating their view completely. This is ineffective and produces poor results.

It's much easier to effectively communicate when the topics are easy to address. But what about the ones that aren't? How do you communicate in a healthy and open way about topics that are complex and even controversial? Let's apply our first core principle and break down how you can effectively communicate about even the most controversial topics to address. At the top of nearly every list, the top common hotly debated controversial topics were related to:

- Gun Control
- Abortion
- Religious Freedom
- Animal Rights
- Vaccines
- Privacy Rights
- Global Climate Change
- Racism
- Sexism
- Capitalism
- Love and Relationships

Typically a topic becomes controversial when someone has competing values and interests. When someone strongly disagrees about statements, assertions, or actions with someone else that touches on some particular sensitivity it arouses an emotional reaction. How could I possibly talk about global climate change with someone if I believe in it and they don't? Why would I want to? Shouldn't I just avoid these topics altogether?

Won't it be triggering or even toxic? You'll discover these answers by the end of this exercise when we take a closer look at what we do, how we do it, and ultimately what our results are no matter what the situation or topic is. Firstly, I want you to make a plan to chat with someone that has a more polarizing view than yours. This doesn't have to be a "Hey (*insert random name here*) can we talk about something that's been on my mind?" It can be as simple as when you are around that person in a natural way and seek out an opportunity to chat about a topic.

Always know the overall desired result you want to have from communicating about a controversial topic. What do you want from the exchange? Do you want to change people's minds? Are you simply informing them? Are you trying to promote a willingness to work together in spite of differences? Are you debunking current myths? When you're clear about your motivations then you'll have a path forward of how you can make the actual change you want to see.

Here are a few more great questions to ask yourself so you're clear on how to address a topic that could be controversial. The following applies to any topic you want to address:

- What will happen / won't happen if I let it go?
- What emotions am I experiencing about this particular topic?
- Why is this conflict important to me?
- What would I be willing to do to resolve it?
- What would a potential resolution look like?
- What would I be willing to accept?
- What won't I accept?
- What does this conflict reveal about me and my values?
- What are my intentions?
- Which of my needs are being neglected?
- Which of my needs are being satisfied by this conflict?
- What do I feel I have gained or lost by this conflict?
- How will a resolution best serve my interests?

Be prepared and make sure you know the subject matter you want to discuss well. If you can, do your homework on that polarizing topic you want to bring up. Consider what information might be difficult for someone to understand and prepare yourself to explain those parts. Think of analogies or short stories to help explain the topic. Always avoid any unnecessary jargon or technical terminology. That can sometimes backfire and make you come across as arrogant or pretentious. It's better to just talk to someone on a simple, human level.

When the time comes for you to have your opportunity to communicate with that person make sure you do it in a neutral setting and ease into the conversation. Always acknowledge and recognize the other person's perspective is their reality and their truth. Ask questions and make statements to learn where that person is coming from.

Take time to ask what preconceived ideas and information that person already has. This allows them to feel as if they have a voice in the conversation. Here are some great questions to learn more about that person, address your concerns/topic, and get the results you're trying to achieve. ground. Here are critical questions you should be asking that will help you with this:

- What characteristic do you most admire in others?
- What kind of impact do you hope to have in the world?
- If I visited the city where you came from, where is the first place you would take me?
- What are some common misconceptions people have about you?
- Where do your beliefs come from? Family? Church? Work?

- What do you think your beliefs might be if you had been born into a different family, religion, race, gender, class, or time?
- What is at the heart of this issue, for you as an individual?
- Why do you care so much about this issue?
- What is it about this topic that concerns you the most?
- Do you see issues or ideas you find difficult to define?
- Do you have any mixed feelings, doubts, uncertainties, or discomforts regarding this issue that you would be willing to share?
- What questions do you have for people who have different views?
- What facts, if proven to be true, might cause you to think differently?
- Would you like to know something that would make this situation work?
- Are you willing to do that next time we talk?
- What made you willing to participate in this conversation?
- What would you like to do differently in the future if we disagree?
- How could we make our dialogue ongoing or more effective?
- Do you think it would be useful to continue this conversation, to learn more from each other and what we each believe to be true?
- What would you be willing to let go of in order to move on?

Whenever you're explaining your own views, be mindful of reframing things to create a different way or perspective from which to view a situation. It might be good to use questions and statements like, "Could there be another way to look at this?", "Consider for a moment that…" "What if…?", or "I'm wondering what message this is sending and how it's being received. Do you think you would have said this/drawn this conclusion if…"

If someone has said something that you found offensive because of their view on a certain matter, always make sure you identify what it is exactly that you found offensive or have a disagreement with. Talk about that directly and politely explain which specific words or phrases you experienced as disrespectful (or that someone else might have). Use an "I" statement to express your feelings, as appropriate, rather than commenting on or labeling anyone. For example, try, "Saying ____ often comes up in popular culture. Some might find it problematic because of ____", "When you said X, I felt like Y. In the future, please…", "This seems like a good time to revisit and remind ourselves about the guidelines for discussion that we agreed upon as class."

During this exchange, it will no doubt be uncomfortable and at times get heated. When that does, just use this time as an opportunity to formulate a strategy for re-engaging the hot moment in a productive, inclusive way at another time. Now, here are some key takeaways from the results we can get from even engaging in effective communication on the most polarizing of topics:

If everything for the most part went smoothly even if it wasn't a comfortable exchange (it won't be). Ask yourself do you feel more empowered by doing this? Or deflated? Did you grow from this exchange or not really at all? Did you achieve the results you were looking for? In any regards, you are growing as a person and an effective communicator just by taking the action to communicate with someone else who shares a different view than your own.

You'll notice that there is more emphasis on you inquiring

about the other person and discovering more about why they hold the views that they do. Why is that? Shouldn't you be giving them the lowdown and straightening them out? Remember, there is much more power in learning, listening, and understanding someone else. It's especially important if it's from someone that holds a different view than yours.

When you're allowing room for someone else to be heard and seen they will trust you more and usually be just as patient with you when you share your thoughts. Some people would disagree with this because they simply don't want to acknowledge or learn anything about someone else. But, we can't learn and make effective changes from any situation unless we're able to grow and understand one another first. This will also provide you the opportunity to be more clear about how you can effectively communicate your views in the future and what you can do better. Just by being intentional about thinking clearly and taking action, you're putting your values, principles, and even purpose to the test in one of the most challenging ways.

You just made yourself stronger in every way possible, inwardly and outwardly. You just got a clear example of how you are showing up in the world. You inadvertently taught a valuable listen to the person you're communicating with. Whether they see things more in your way or they're just as committed to their views as before. Something did change for both of you. Let's say you tried out this little exercise of ours and it went poorly.

The other person was non-compliant or worse this whole situation escalated into a heated exchange and your game plan went out the goddamn window. Now, you're even more uncomfortable and pissed about the situation (and that person). That could happen. That person could even get more combative or undermine every point you make.

Perhaps with every question you ask, they are unresponsive. Maybe the more you're trying to communicate in a healthy way, the more they attack you, and see that as a weakness. I've dealt with this from my own personal experiences. I faced off with an executive whom I actually helped in hiring in the first place. He undermined me repeatedly and I experienced these really weird micro-aggressions that it became abundantly clear I had to say something. I tried the above tactics I laid out for you. When we spoke about this uncomfortable topic he remained calm about the whole thing. To my surprise he even apologized. But his behavior never changed.

In fact, it became worse. I didn't take it personally though. It became clear that whatever he was doing wasn't about me. It was about him. I was proud that I handled the situation in the way I knew to be true to who I was as a person.

It even made me more confident about my beliefs, values, and overall the way I handled the situation. So, that specific situation didn't improve but it did help improve the way I dealt with other situations. When you try new ways to improve your life and they "don't work " do not see it as a waste of time. It's not. Instead ask yourself what lessons did you learn about yourself and what could you have done better?

It's never a waste and it's never a loss when you attempt to make a situation better and you do it with clarity of thought. Let's say someone stays combative or they undermine every point you make and every question you ask, they are unresponsive. In fact, the more you're trying to communicate in a healthy way the more they attack you and see that as a weakness. The fact that you remained steady and in integrity with yourself, you always win. Now, once you've done this.

Do it again. With the same person, about the same topic or find someone or something else to find ways to continue effective communication. In the end, there are no losers in this. It's a win-win. Always follow up with a "check in" after your conversations.

Let them know that you value their experiences and perspective. You should especially revisit something said or did that caught you by surprise or a missed opportunity that you wish you could have a do-over in response to a micro-aggression or "hot moment". Even if the moment has passed, it's ok to go back and address it late. Research actually indicates that an unaddressed micro-aggression can leave just as much of a negative impact as the micro-aggression itself. If you're not sure how to address it. Try something like, "I want to go back to something that was brought up in our last conversation" or "I think it would be worthwhile to revisit something that happened ____."

Good communication improves relationships, minimizes distractions, and improves your overall quality of life. This is the type of challenging action that doesn't just transform your life it transforms others.

CHAPTER FOUR

Can You Leash Your Dog?

Asking the right questions isn't a luxury. We live in a time where the wrong choice at the wrong time can quickly turn you into a viral sensation for all of the wrong reasons. All because you didn't just take a beat to ask the right questions. Human beings are emotional creatures first and intelligent second. We use our decision-making choices in life strictly out of emotional responses for pleasure, pain, safety, and joy. This has to be your way of life for you to thrive in our world.

What happens if you don't take out the time to ask the right questions? What can happen if you don't take out the time to reflect and understand your place in the world? This can be answered in the true cautionary tale of Amy and Christian Cooper (unrelated).

On the morning of May 25th, 2020, Amy Cooper walked her dog in an area of Central Park known as the "Ramble." Amy Cooper was a successful businesswoman who lived in New York City. She was well known in her community for regularly volunteering to help watchdogs that needed a loving home. The Central Park Conservancy requires that dogs in that part of the park be on a leash. On this particular day, Amy decided not to leash her dog. This did not go unnoticed and local birdwatcher Christian Cooper approached Amy.

Christian asked Amy to leash her dog. She refused. Christian said by his own account, "Look, if you're going to do what you want, I'm going to do what I want. But you're not going to like it." Then he beckoned the dog toward him with a treat. What happens next is a clear example of how bias, poor judgment, and a lack of clarity can make small choices have even larger outcomes.

Before we continue on, we need to understand the full context of the situation. The "ramble" requires dog owners to leash their dogs because it's an area of Central Park that is a natural preservation habitat for birds. Unleashed dogs have a history of attacking and killing birds. There are signs everywhere, even stating this. Because of its location, it is also quite common for bird watchers to be in the area.

"Birdwatchers" identify birds and understand what they are doing in their natural habitat. They are also known to preserve the safety of the birds in their habitat. So it's not uncommon for one to request a dog owner to leash their dog if one is unleashed. The most crucial detail of this story is to also know that Amy Cooper is a white woman. Christian Cooper is a Black man. Upon Christian's request to leash her dog, Amy yelled back in response, "Don't you touch my dog!"

The video begins with Amy charging at Christian, asking him to stop recording and pointing her finger in his face. He responds with, *"Please don't come close to me."* Amy angrily boils and threatens Christian, "I'm calling the cops … I'm gonna tell them there's an African American man threatening my life." At this moment, anyone who's seen this video is dumbfounded that

Amy chose to knowingly put a man's life at risk by weaponizing the term "African American man." Christian smartly recorded the rest of this exchange on his cell phone, so there's no debate about what happens next.

The entire time that this exchange is happening, Amy is wielding her leash in her hand, and at any time, she could have simply leashed her dog (which is what she was supposed to do). She was also gripping her dog's collar with her dog attached. So, it would appear that Amy was really losing her shit. Amy then makes good on her threat and calls the police.

When connected to a 9-1-1 operator, she says, "There is an African American man—I am in Central Park— he is recording me and threatening myself and my dog. Please send the cops immediately!"

Instead of simply diffusing the situation, Amy attempted to manipulate the police and threaten a man's life… because he asked her to leash her dog… which was the law. Christian's recording finally ends when Amy reluctantly leashes her dog. Christian thanks her and goes on his way.

Why did Amy, a seasoned dog owner who has obviously walked in this area before, decide not to leash her dog this one time? If there was one person who should know to leash her dog, it's Amy. If only she had taken a moment to check her ego and question her entitlement, she could have easily avoided this situation. Perhaps she could acknowledge the truth of the situation, "Do I need to leash my dog?" Amy had so many choices to choose from. She decided to escalate the situation.

Like I said before, human beings are emotional creatures. It is a common misconception that we can separate our emotions from our decision-making. Even when we are thinking clearly, our choices are influenced by emotion. In the case of Amy Cooper, one could surmise that based on her principles and values, she felt embarrassed, angry, and even threatened by Christian's attempt to check her.

The story isn't over, though. This was actually just the beginning of a national firestorm. This exchange happened at the beginning stages of the global Covid-19 pandemic when everyone was glued to their screens, absorbing everything and anything. Christian Cooper's sister posted a video of the incident on her Twitter account. It instantly went viral. The Twitter video alone received over 40 million views at the time.

Amy's response to Christian was rightfully criticized for falsely presenting herself as being in immediate physical danger and conjuring a checkered history of exploiting the tendency for racial bias with immediate suspicion. Amy's employer, Franklin Templeton, viewed the video, then placed her on administrative leave pending an investigation. The following day, the company fired her from her position as head of the firm's insurance investment.

Even those who were not shaken by Amy's response to Christian were deeply disturbed by her violently dragging her dog by its collar. That incident alone forced her to have to surrender her dog to the shelter from which she had adopted him two years prior. On June 3rd, after an evaluation by the shelter's veterinarian, the dog was returned to Amy.

Amy Cooper unknowingly became a part of history by becoming the perfect amalgamation of exhibit A in "white privilege", "playing the race card", "woman in distress", and being "Karen" (a relatively new term for a typically white woman who appears to be entitled or demanding beyond the scope of what is normal).

The Amy Cooper incident even re-ignited a previously introduced legislative bill to the state of New York. This bill considers falsely reporting criminal incidents against protected groups of people, including race, gender, and religion, to be a hate crime. Violators can face prison time if the motivation for reporting such crime is motivated by a perception or belief about their race, color, national origin, ancestry, gender, religion, religious practice, age, disability, or sexual orientation.

The bill was signed into law in June 2020, piggybacking off the Cooper situation. Even the Central Park Civic Association asked New York City Mayor Bill de Blasio to ban Amy from the park. Amy was also charged with filing a false police report. But it would be Christian Cooper who declined to cooperate with enforcement officials. He expanded on his feelings in a Washington Post op-ed piece, saying he was ambivalent about prosecuting her because "I think it's a mistake to focus on this one individual. The incident highlights the importance of the long-standing, deep-seated racial bias against us black and brown folk that permeates the United States."

Coincidentally something else happened on the day of the Cooper situation. The death of George Floyd. The outpouring of emotions from these two incidents alone didn't just impact the United States. It affected the global landscape. Amy could have avoided all the drama and becoming a headline for all the wrong reasons by simply asking herself better questions to get a grip on reality.

Christian disrupted Amy's reality. From her perspective, Amy was a victim who was defending herself from an attack. You can clearly see it's no easy feat to disrupt your reality even if you're facing the facts of a situation. When we dig deeper to see what was happening with Amy Cooper, we can also understand how the ego works against us and how it can be a cousin to unconscious bias. I'm sure you have been in a situation where you overacted or acted out of character.

After all, we're human. I'm sure we have all felt a bit embarrassed about that, responding in different ways. Whether that's learning how to respond better, pretending it didn't happen, or doubling down on it. This is deeply rooted in our identities, values, and how we perceive the world we live in. It's a lot easier said than done when faced with the realities of our day-to-day challenges.

This is why you need to practice asking better questions. To question your feelings appropriately. It only takes a moment for you to pause. You have to practice this if it's foreign to you. Get into the habit of reframing your perspective. When we reframe, we ask better questions and even, at times, discover painful answers. Remember that emotional pain is a part of the human process. We have increasingly gotten more comfortable being in safe bubbles. All bubbles burst.

More often than not, we say we don't have time to check in with ourselves. In reality, there's a hidden reason why we don't. It's simply that it's not a top priority. Perhaps, we're scared that we might stumble onto hard truths we're not ready for, and that gamble is a terrifying one to take. Again, when your reality is challenged, that disrupts your entire identity. Your body and mind subconsciously do things to protect you from the truth without you even knowing.

Accept that pain is a part of life. Through reflection and action, we find progress in it. Choose to take into account your principles, boundaries, and values. The reality of who you are and what you're about. There can be no confusion about how you respond in life when you know who you are in life. Continuously check in with yourself and update your priorities as you evolve in life. Always ask yourself if a situation, regardless of how you feel, matches up with your core values. After all, every moment, you're evolving and changing.

Even after the myriad of consequences, Amy Cooper received, both she and Christian Cooper never spoke since the incident in Central Park. In fact, only a year later, in August 2021, Amy said on the podcast, *Honestly with Bari Weiss* about her encounter with Christian, "I'd explored all my options. I tried to leave. I tried to look for anyone who's around", she recalled. As to why she called the police, she added, "There was no noise, no sound. And it was, you know, it was my last attempt to sort of hope that he would step down and leave me alone." When asked what she would say to Christian if she had the opportunity, Amy responded, "The one that really, I really would just like to start and open this conversation with is, 'You scared me.'"

In the stories we tell ourselves, everyone has to be the hero, and someone has to be the villain. In Amy's reality, she has chosen to still be the hero. Even more so, she feels that she was a victim even though the reality of the situation proved otherwise. This is why we have to dismantle the stories we tell ourselves and question everything.

CHAPTER FIVE

Why Did We Break Up?

Nothing is more relatable to disrupting one's reality than going through a tough breakup. There are an estimated 7.8 billion people on the planet. The average global life expectancy is now 70 years. At 365 days per year, that amounts to 25,567 days. It's expected that everyone on this planet goes through at least two breakups in their lifetime. At two significant breakups per person's lifetime, that would amount to a total of 13.6 billion breakups across the lifespans of everyone on our planet. So if you think your world is crashing in on you from an excruciating breakup, stop and realize that 531,024 others are suffering the same fate every day.

In our society, there are certain expectations when you're in a loving and committed relationship. After all, you and your partner have dreamed of infinite possibilities. When it all falls apart, it's brutal. No matter how many phone calls, texts, meetups, make-up sessions, arguments… there ain't no going back. This doesn't just fuck up your life. It destroys your reality.

The story you built up in your head about what was supposed to happen has crumbled away. Ultimately, this is a turning point in our lives that will change how we view ourselves and the world around us moving forward.

When a couple goes through a tough breakup, the brain experiences massive withdrawal symptoms almost identical to a heroin addict quitting cold turkey. You should expect withdrawal symptoms and increase your self-care and social support during this season. If you and your partner have broken up, it's only natural to wonder how long it'll take for your feelings of love toward them to fade. There is no standard timeline if you will. Not all relationships end poorly either. In some cases, there may still be a lot of love between the people in the relationship. There is no wrong or correct answer.

Then there is another layer of complexity and challenge that comes from breakups through the lens of social media and our digital lives. When you experience a split now, it isn't just people you know in real life that notice. It's also your digital life too. This has caused so much anxiety for people that so many of us hide the status of our relationships or are even ambiguous about who we are dating just in case it doesn't work out. Even more than that, it helps avoid putting unneeded pressure and relationships under a microscope.

I experienced this first-hand when I dealt with a life-changing breakup. This was after my divorce, and I dated someone whom I felt was my soulmate, and we were also in sync professionally. Both business partners and lovers, we were inseparable. Couple goals. We had this unique rhythm of understanding each other so well, and we would dream together. Even more impressive, we would help each other realize our dreams. I couldn't see my life without her. When we finally did break up, my life came to a crashing halt.

Unbinding our lives was a constant headache and trigger. I decided to lean into my career, especially using my professional skills as a growth marketer and my creative skills to my advantage. This is where I embraced my journey as an "Influencer". I wanted to reshape my identity and universe completely. It worked. Outwardly, it seemed like I lived the perfect life. Inwardly, however, I was still experiencing an existential crisis and battling depression while trying to discover my new identity.

The world can feel especially cruel during a breakup because as you try to pause and recenter yourself, the world keeps spinning. Life goes on with or without you. At the time of our break up, the world was rapidly changing around us. Digital and in-person lives became more intertwined to the point that my tough earth-shattering breakup became a constant game of understanding what was real and what wasn't. It got increasingly more complex and bizarre each passing day as my personal life and work dealt directly with social media. It was unavoidable. When I logged onto Facebook, my entire body became so tense that I had to stop logging in altogether. It took another two years before I updated my relationship status.

Then there was Instagram which at the time declared they would shift their algorithmic feed to what it thought you would like versus content in chronological order. One day, I looked at my suggested feed, and nearly all of the photos were of my ex. It was like each picture was a different snapshot of how extraordinary her life was. She and I used the same photo editing filters and shot composition, so essentially the Instagram algorithm said, "Oh, you take photos like these, so we think you would like this a lot."

I had an anxiety attack and even threw up afterward. I was already struggling with an overwhelming depression from our breakup. This stung even more. I could clearly see how happy she was. Not just happy, thriving while I was suffering. How could this be?

The truth is we all have a tendency to make up narratives in our own heads based on our own life experiences. A lot of the stories we tell ourselves are untrue. We tend to project those false narratives, especially online. We can debate with each other on which one matters the most, but we should be able to agree that we need to challenge the false narratives that we're projecting onto each other. It's negatively reshaping expectations and causing more harm than good.

This brings me back to my breakup. I was hell-bent on focusing on self-improvement and healing my mind, body, and soul. I also really leaned into my support system of family, friends, and colleagues. I was even joined by one of my best friends, who began helping me as a creative partner. It's important to point out that my friend is a lingerie model, and although our relationship was platonic, it would be easy to assume we were dating.

The truth is that she was going through a rough breakup of her own. We helped each other heal while we were gassing each other up. She was like my sister. Eventually, when we did find new romantic partners, we were private about it without the pressures of social media. So, essentially no one ever saw who they were actually dating. Which is another reason why you shouldn't assume anything.

Later in life, my ex and I would reconnect. I discovered in our conversations that most of what I thought to be true wasn't the case at all. She was hurt and just as depressed about our breakup as I was. Even more shocking was that from her perspective, she was having trouble understanding how I was so much happier, healthier, and living my best life when she was struggling. We were both wrong about our assumptions and the stories we told ourselves. We just made up stories in our own minds.

The reality, though, was that we were just two people in pain from a breakup, and we just wanted to re-discover ourselves. As I said, each of us has our own sense of reality. In the case of a split, every one of us will respond differently. Some of us will jump right into a new relationship. Some of us will do the opposite. When it comes to our online lives, no one will truly see the pain you're going through from a breakup. Not really.

You will undoubtedly ask yourself questions to make sense of things. You're going to ask yourself, your family, friends, co-workers, strangers, and hell, even your ex. Typically, you'll ask the wrong types of questions that can quickly put you in an endless cycle of psychological and physical turmoil. There isn't anything wrong with this. You are grieving, and this is a process. But we can always make the process better. Remember what I stated before.

We do want to question everything, but we do it to empower ourselves, not to shit on ourselves. There's a difference. See for yourself. Below are the most common questions we ask ourselves right after a breakup. DO NOT ask these questions:

- Why don't they care that we broke up?
- What's wrong with me?
- What did I do wrong?
- How can I fix this?
- Will we get back together?
- Was my ex cheating on me?
- Are all men/women like this?

- Should I just move on or hold out for my ex to come back?
- Why don't they love me?
- What can I do to win them back?
- This was obviously a mistake. How can we fix this mistake?
- Why can't they see things the way I do?
- Did they ever love me in the first place?
- What could I have done differently?

These questions, while they are common and to be expected, can put you in a tailspin of misery and overthinking if you're not careful. Your mind is trying to find a new story to tell yourself about why the original story you told yourself has evaporated. But, these questions put you in a position of helplessness and weakness. You're giving away all of your power. The worst part is that you're creating more challenges for yourself that aren't really there.

Instead of asking those types of questions, what would be better questions to ask ourselves? Take a look and see how these questions feel in comparison to our previous questions:

- Why would I want to be with someone that doesn't want to be with me?
- Now that they are out of the picture (at least for the time being), what have I been missing out on since being with them?
- What is something simple I can do for myself that makes me happy?
- What was my role in the demise of this relationship?
- What can I do differently in my next relationship?
- Have I been realistic in my expectations?

- Would I date myself?
- What is my limiting belief?
- What are three lessons I learned from being with this person?
- Did they make me a better person?
- If so, how can I continue these habits without them?
- Where have I been neglecting my own self-compassion?
- Who do I want to be in my next relationship?
- What are the healthy things I'm doing to support myself during my breakup?

How did it feel when you answered these questions instead of the previous ones? Did you sense the difference? If you notice, the better questions tie into supporting you in discovering a new sense of identity post-breakup in a positive way. Most importantly, the questions are aimed at what you can control. Not what you can't.

You cannot force anyone to love you. Asking why someone doesn't love you back is irrelevant. Why you choose to love someone that doesn't love you back is. When you ask better questions aimed at self-awareness and your own agency in the situation, you will ultimately find new ways to improve your own life. Don't reach for the questions that will make you stagnant or, worse, feel less about yourself and others.

If there is much power in asking better questions to oneself, one could easily surmise that there is merit in asking better questions to people in your life. Not only does asking better questions provide you with more insight, but it also provides you with more opportunities for success and happiness. We learn and grow from asking questions. Never stop asking questions.

Before you discover *The Maguire Method's* second principle, take out some time to answer the following questions for yourself. Ask them aloud. Write down your answers. Keep them with you to reference whenever you need to:

- What am I grateful for?
- What drives me more… my ego or my purpose?
- Has caring about others' opinions propelled me forward or held me back?
- What will people say about me at my funeral?
- Which do I REALLY think is worse for me: failing or never trying?
- When it's all said and done, will I have said more than I've done?
- Is it more important to love or be loved?
- If this were the last day of my life, would I want to do what I am about to do today?
- Am I holding on to something I need to let go of?
- What am I doing about the things that matter most in my life?
- Have I made someone smile today?
- What small act of kindness was I once shown that I will never forget?

REFLECTIONS

PRINCIPLE II

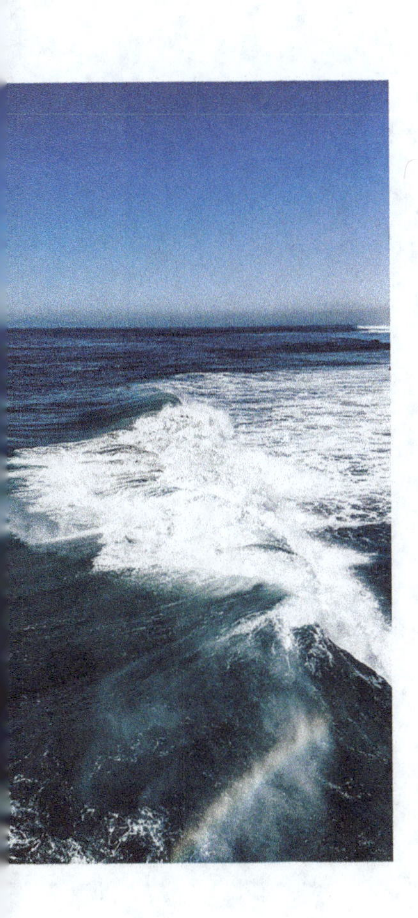

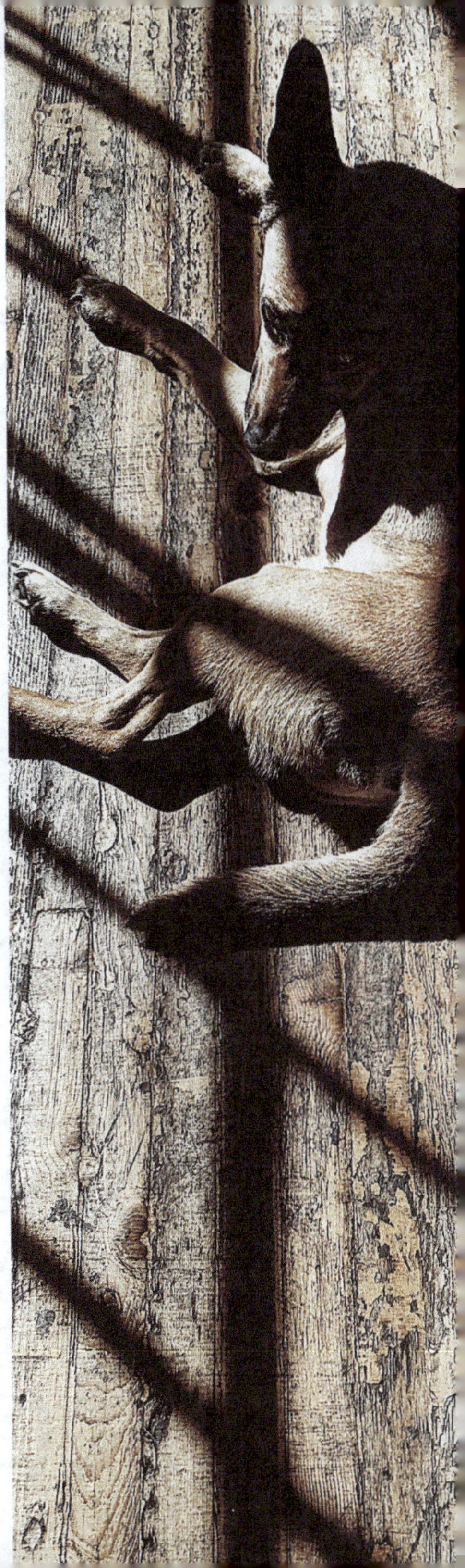

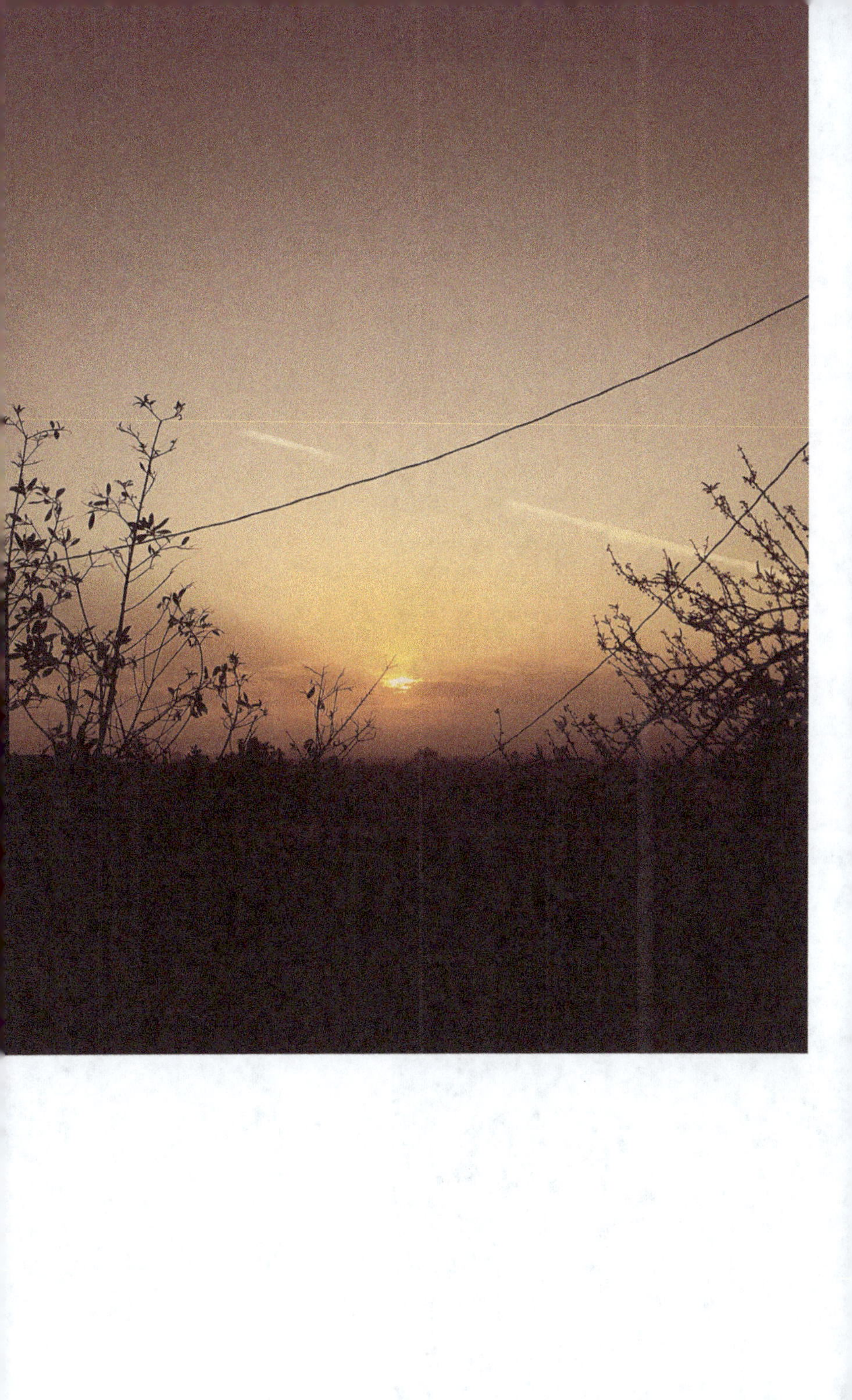

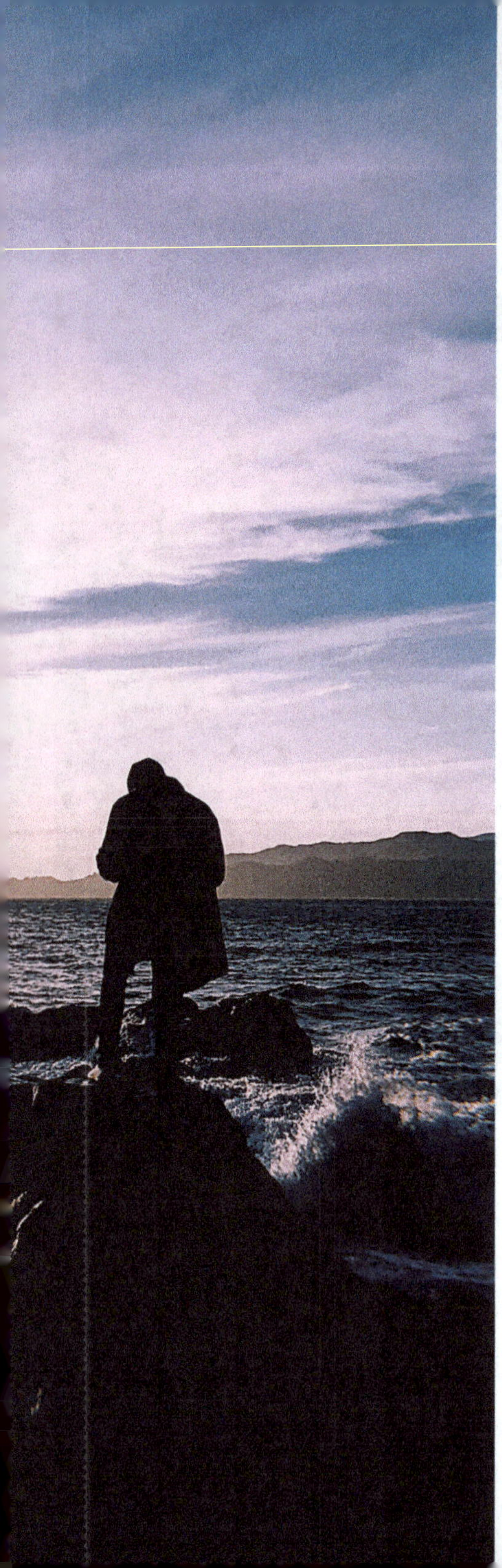

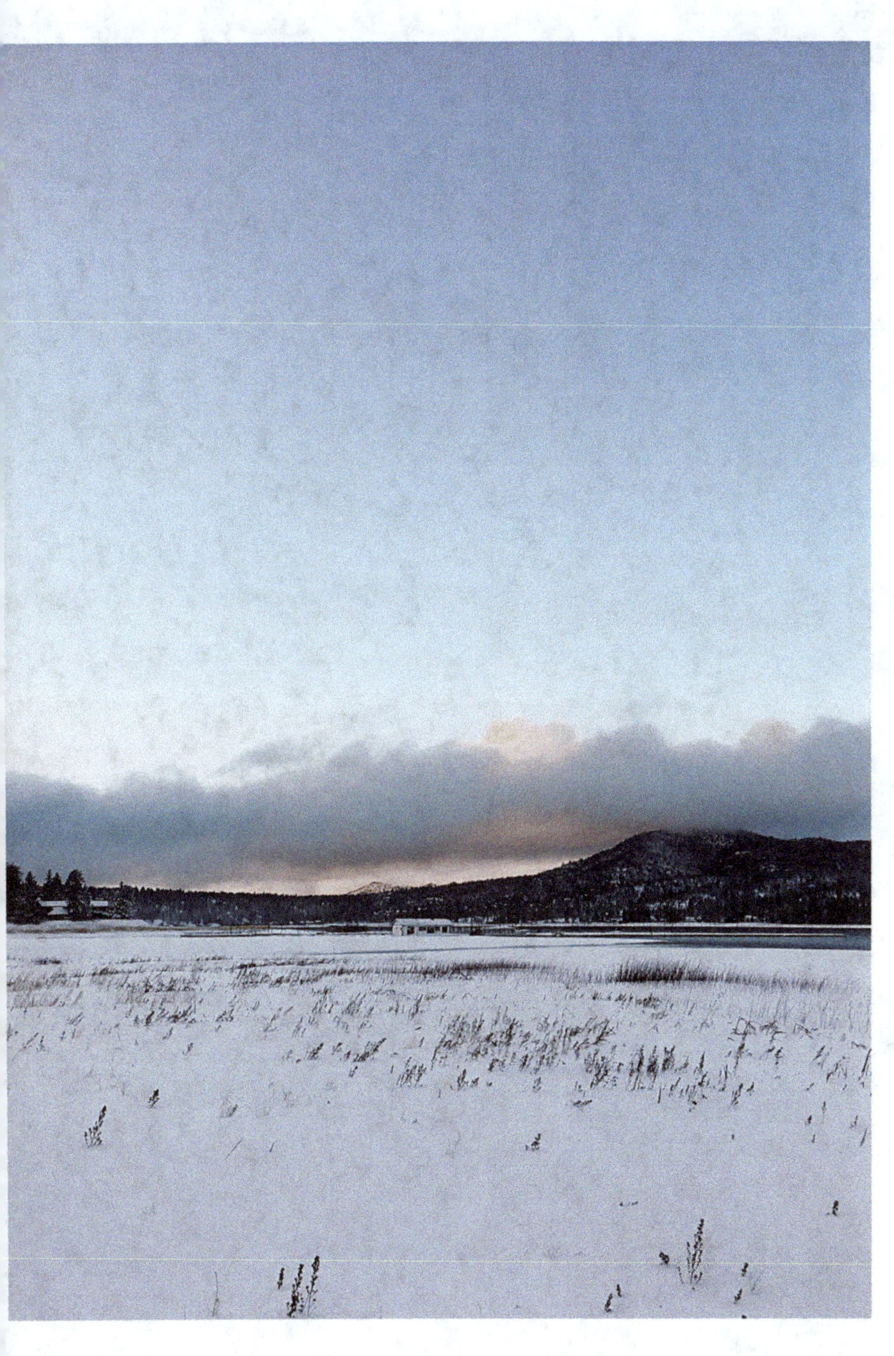

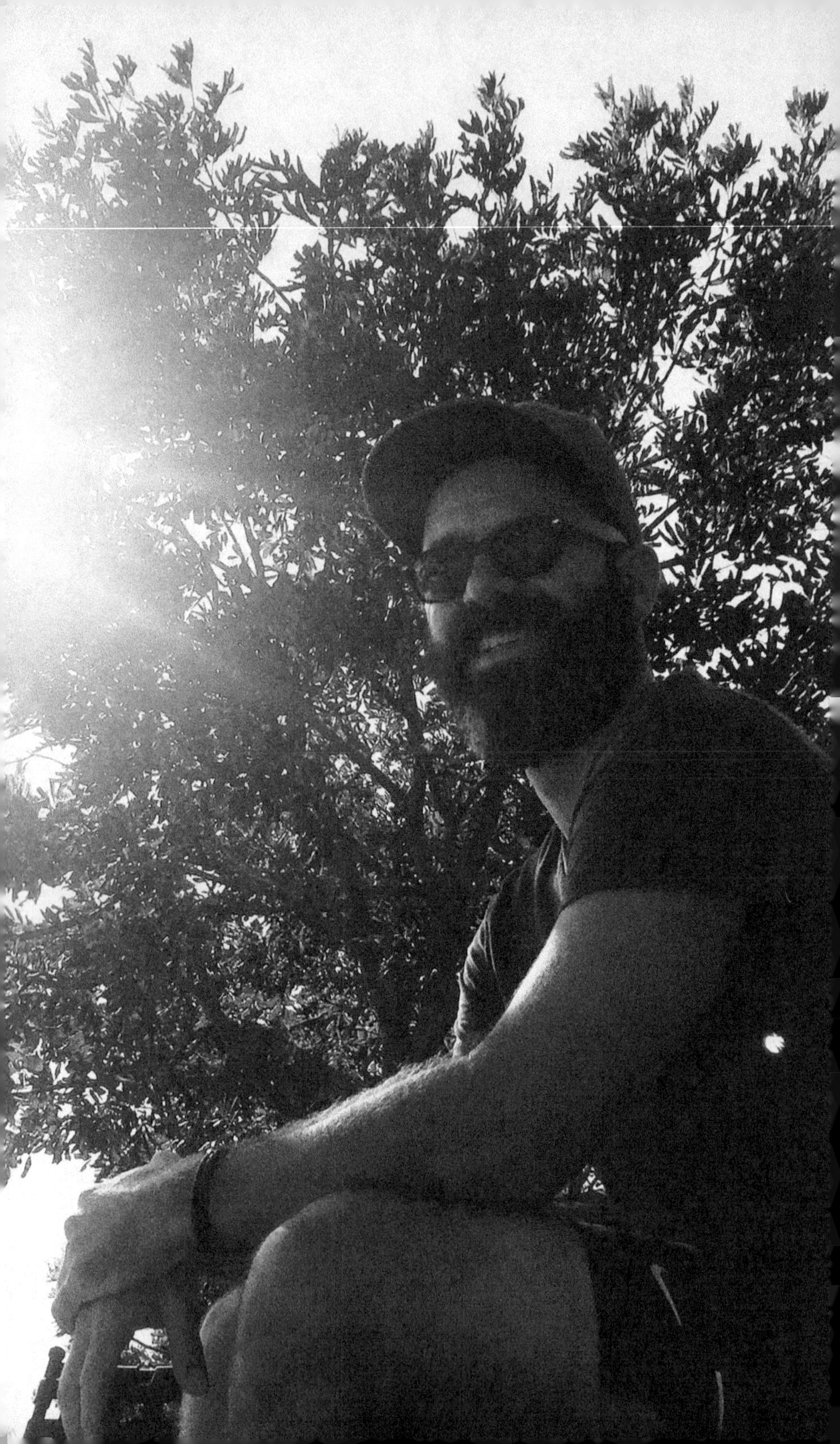

CHAPTER SIX

The Discovery of Purpose

Reflections – this is our second principle and the most challenging and rewarding one. Reflection gives the brain an opportunity to pause amidst the chaos of our mind and the world around us. We use reflection as a way to sort through observations and experiences, consider multiple possible interpretations, and create meaning to our lives. This meaning becomes learning, which can then inform future mindsets and actions.

When we reflect, we gain more insights of ourselves to further learn about our strengths, weaknesses, fears, and might even discover something unexpected. In the times that we live in now, it's more critical than ever to invest more of our time and ourselves into reflecting. Reflection is our second principle because simply put, when you ask a question, it directly leads to reflection. These two principles work hand in hand. To reflect in a sense is to be self-aware, and to be self-aware is liberating.

Reflection is the one thing you can do alone that answers many questions for yourself, including your purpose, reality, and identity. Reflection can be taken literally. I've often faced myself in the mirror to understand my own purpose and the reality of my world. Reflection leads to self-awareness, which, as we learned earlier, is a direct confrontation with your reality. If you discover yourself to be right about things you thought to be true, it's validating and empowering.

If you find out you're wrong, then it's painful but that pain is always necessary for growth. There are many certainties in life. One is that you *will* experience pain at some point in your life. You must have the courage to face your suffering directly as too many people stifle themselves all in the name of avoiding pain, which is nothing we can truly outrun. Through pain, there is progress. Finding true significance and purpose from pain is something that human beings have been striving to embrace since the birth of our existence.

It is genuinely through acknowledging the pain that we can reflect in the first place. This is much more difficult to acknowledge and face now because we have so many distractions at our disposal that pull us away from looking inward. These distractions from our bond with our mobile devices to social media is typically the reason why reflection is the most challenging part of our method. After all, you're asking yourself to use your free will to actively and consciously pursue the very thing your mind is evolutionarily trained to avoid. Our ancestors didn't outrun sabretooth tigers by stopping to acknowledge discomfort, pain, and fear.

Yet in today's world, when we face things head-on and reflect on the meaning, it actually saves us time and ultimately may prevent further or repetitive pain in the future. It has been said that you are our own worst enemy. If that were true, it also means you are your own best ally.

There will always be external factors in life that are entirely out of our control that can really fuck us up. But the truth is that we often don't look at how things happen *for* us. I will say this again clearly. Things do not happen *to* you. They happen *for* you. Realize and embrace this notice, and you already have a tool that most do not. Even under the most stressful, bizarre, and awful experiences, there are lessons to be learned.

When bad things happen to us, it hurts so much that we try to discover the significance of why we feel the pain in the first place. Whatever it is, no matter how painful it is, always follow the first step of asking good questions. Don't ask "Why me?" Ask yourself what is the lesson that you can learn from the experience. There is no better story to serve as a great example of discovering growth and meaning through pain than the story of Viktor E. Frankl. A Holocaust survivor who truly experienced and witnessed first-hand the atrocities of evil men.

He witnessed his own family murdered. His first wife died in a concentration camp. He was forced to do hard labor under extreme physical conditions (starvation, cold, filth, etc). He endured years of emotional, physical, and mental torture. If there was one person who had every excuse to give up or to let the pain wash over him, it was Viktor.

Yet he did something quite remarkable. After his horrific experiences, he reflected on the traumas he endured. He would go on to write *The Man's Search For Meaning*, a book in which he details the nightmarish horrors he faced and discovers a life's purpose from it all. His book is considered one of the top 10 most influential books in the United States and has been listed in countless Top 100 lists worldwide.

Sometimes, especially during difficult times, I think about what he went through in his life. How everything he envisioned for himself and his life was stripped away from him within a blink of an eye. I think about the times I ignored texts and calls from my friends. I think about how I get annoyed when my sister complains about dating, or my mom goes on and on about the crazy world we live in. But I couldn't imagine any of them being prosecuted, rounded up, and killed in front of me. Moreover, it's difficult to see how any of us would experience *that* and then proceed to find a silver lining.

It's hard not to think of that lumped in with other historical atrocities. The ugliness of it all. I myself, a descendant of African slaves, targeted at times consciously and - equally disturbing - unconsciously just for the shade of my skin. When you reflect on the painful traumas or challenges you face, think of the story of Viktor E. Frankl. Put things into perspective of how he would go on to love again. To live again. To dare to thrive after facing pure evil and a dark abyss of unwavering pain.

Even survivors of abuse can use the tragedies they once faced to be a voice for the voiceless. A great example of this is one of the all-time greatest poets to ever live, Maya Angelou. She used her voice to bring hope, joy, and liberty to the oppressed and marginalized. Her childhood was fraught with painful events. Her parents divorced.

She and her siblings were sent to live with relatives. She suffered sexual abuse at the age of seven. Her abuser was arrested and later murdered after being released from prison. This experience made her mute, believing that it was her voice that killed the man who abused her. Growing up, she worked in the nightclub district as a sex worker.

Maya Angelou would go on to marry twice, with both marriages ending in failure. Through it all, she held onto her passion for the written word, and her literary works were eventually recognized internationally. The strength she possessed allowed her to go through all the difficulties in her life. She would eventually become an inspiration to many who are fighting for their rights even today.

We must find meaning in our lives even through the darkest of times. Despite your beliefs, sex, nationality, or income level, each and every one of us wants our life to have meaning. Meaning is the emotional significance of what we do. It's why we do what we do. It doesn't just exist on its own. It's something that we have to create and feel. Our life's purpose is the cumulative effect of our meaning.

In the most straightforward way, we have to first ask ourselves, "What do I want?" It sounds simple enough. However, what I've discovered through a personal and professional lens, it's the question that most of us have difficulty answering. Even if we always have the answer. We just need to look inward. Philosopher Alan Watts once stated the following, "You don't know what you want. Because one, you already have it. Or two, you don't know yourself."

We have to discover ourselves in a real way. That's where Reflection plays a significant role. Reflection transforms thoughts into genuine learning about how our beliefs and values affect happiness, life choices and goal achievement. Understanding how your beliefs and values affect you is the first step towards uncovering your life's purpose. Discovering your purpose is part of the whole journey of life. This is not just an intellectual pursuit or even something tied to your career. Finding your purpose in life might sound like a nice-to-have, but it's more important than you may think.

Having a purpose is an essential tool for a better, happier, and ultimately healthier life for yourself. Around 25% of American adults cite having a clear sense of purpose. While 40% were neutral on the subject or said they don't have one at all. Your life purpose consists of the central motivating aims of your life. It's the reason why you get up in the morning.

Living a purpose driven life contributes to better physical health and mental fitness. It also reduces the risk of chronic disease. Multiple studies have even found that it can help you live longer. Having a sense of purpose comes from feeling connected to others. Using your gifts and skills in the service of others can help you find your true purpose, while isolation and loneliness can cause you to have an existential crisis.

You will probably find that your purpose changes throughout your life. Continuous growth and progress can help you stay connected to your purpose. Purpose can guide life decisions, influence behavior, shape goals, offer a sense of direction, and create meaning. For some people, purpose is connected to meaningful, satisfying work. For example, you might discover "My life purpose is to stand up for issues that I believe in and to contribute positively to my community. I want to leave the world knowing that I made it a better place."

This would mean that you find a strong sense of purpose from family, consider a statement like this. So, in this case, you would ask yourself how you are personally fulfilled through family, and what you want your life to look like. Another example is more career focused, "My life purpose is to find success in my career. I would like to be a notable person among my peers and be valued for my contributions to my field. My hope is that I will retire feeling fulfilled with what I have accomplished." In this case, you find happiness through achieving success and contributing to society.

So, it would be helpful to specify the particular field, the goals you may have, and why your career gives you a sense of purpose. Or maybe it's just you, being honest, open, and living your own truth, "The purpose of my life is to be my true self, uninhibited by fear. I want to inspire others to live authentically and with passion." You would discover your purpose here by questioning what your passions are and how they empower you. Having a sense of purpose comes from feeling connected to others.

Using your gifts in the service of others can help you find your true purpose, while isolation and loneliness can cause you to have an existential crisis. When you change over time, as we all do in life, so does your purpose. It simply depends on what your values, principles, and boundaries are. If you're true to that, then you are being honest to yourself.

You can use the power of reflection to both discover and even rediscover your purpose. Remember, reflection is a process of exploring and examining ourselves, our perspectives, attributes, experiences, and actions. It helps us gain insight and see how to move forward. Make sure your true inner self knows that your life purpose is out of sync with your outer life. The latter is often a false self, but you've identified with it because it's been so rewarding to your ego. It doesn't matter if you're in a thriving career or stuck in life, connecting with your purpose will always work to your benefit.

You can uncover (or recover your purpose) by trying the following steps:

1. Develop a growth mindset. Having a growth mindset is linked to having a sense of purpose.
2. Create a personal vision statement with a growth mindset. Having a growth mindset is often linked to discovering one's purpose in life.
3. Give back and contribute to others. Seek out opportunities for this with your loved ones and even strangers.
4. Practice gratitude. You'll see this often because it is such a powerful way to reframe things and keep you inspired, putting things into a different perspective.
5. Turn your pain into purpose. From our suffering we can take even the most devastating experiences and learn from them, molding them into sage wisdom we can share with others.
6. Explore your passions. It doesn't matter how big or small your passions are, take the time out to explore them. This will provide you with more fulfillment and clarity.
7. Be part of a community. You will discover throughout this book how important being a part of a community is critical to your own wellbeing.

Use reflection to grow and stay connected to your purpose. Reflecting helps you to develop your skills and review their effectiveness, rather than just carry on doing things as you have always done them. It is about questioning, in a positive way, what you do and why you do it and then deciding whether there is a better, or more efficient, way of doing it in the future.

I discovered at one point in my life my purpose was to provide motivation to others. I never considered myself a guru, and I wasn't necessarily interested in giving inspirational speeches or any of that. I simply wanted to offer a bit of perspective and inspiration for anyone who might need it to help make their dreams a reality. I thought I would be doing it through my creative passions in film or television. I eventually navigated through art school in Los Angeles, and soon after, I became a Video Editor at Mattel Toys.

It was a well-known Fortune 500 company, and I hated every minute of being there. I was stuck in a cubicle or an editing bay, slogging away at creating and digitizing the company's first video library of commercials, trailers, and sizzle reels. At one point, I memorized the airing dates of every single Barbie commercial ever broadcasted. In case you were wondering, the very first Barbie commercial aired in 1959. Every day, I did various assignments and dealt with executives and team leaders from each department. If you think working at a toy company would be fun, you would be correct in that assumption. That would be the building next door to my building. I was in the not so fun corporate environment filled with office gossip, social climbing, and department rivalries that, up until that point, I had only seen in movies.

Outside of that 9-5 slog, I pursued my creative passions in writing, producing, and directing. It was tough to juggle. Exhausting really. I always needed an outlet to blow off steam. As it so happened, photography was the hobby I picked up to do just that. Social media was a fantastic new way to promote my work on my own. Eventually, I was laid off from that corporate job I hated so much. Just like that, my cushy corporate job was whisked away from me.

With a major life event like this happening I was terrified at the uncertainty of it all. After all, this security blanket that I had for so long was tossed aside. More than that though, I took this as an opportunity that life was offering me. I was no longer bound by the mundane tasks of a corporate world and now I had the space to really see how my creative endeavors aligned with my overall purpose. I asked myself questions about what I really wanted in life and my career.

I took the time to reflect on the answers I was coming up with. Life persisted though with the realities and challenges of the real world. I bounced around a lot doing freelance gigs here and there just to keep up with my financial responsibilities of adulting. Meanwhile, I continued sharpening my vision of my real pursuits.

I used the power of reflection to take my accumulated skills and make them work for me to feed my overall purpose, eventually leading me to where I am now. When it all clicked, the journey I took made more sense when I thought about it. The skills I learned being a professional Video Editor had a direct impact on the quality of my creative passions. I already understood the rhythm of tight deadlines, quarterly reports, and assignments, all while working closely with top-level executives. I understood what ineffective and effective leadership looked like up close.

It became abundantly clear the more digging I did that what I took for granted was actually helping me achieve my goals. There are so many great ways you can use to help you thrive with reflection. You do not have to do it alone. That might be therapy for some people who are suffering to the point where you need professional help. It might look like a family member, friend, co-worker, or mentor to someone else. It could even be as simple as speaking aloud to yourself.

Speaking out loud forces us to slow down our thoughts and

process them differently by engaging the language centers of our brain. You can use an audio note on your phone, computer, stroll outside, or around your home just to talk to yourself out loud. Reflecting helps you to develop your skills and review their effectiveness, rather than just carry on doing things as you have always done them. It is about questioning (which is why this is our first core principle), in a positive way. You have to be much more intentional about what you do and why you do it and then decide whether there is a better, or more efficient, way of doing it in the future.

When we fail to reflect on our lives, it limits us from understanding what we are creating and putting out into the world. We lose perspective, get caught up in things that don't matter, and often lose sight of the things that are most important. This leaves us vulnerable to our conditioning, which can include implicit biases as well as limited storylines about what is happening.

CHAPTER SEVEN

The Discovery of Growth

You should always have a safe place to express your thoughts freely. Seek opportunities for growth when you're using reflection. Reflection is often done as writing, possibly because this allows us to probe our reflections and develop them more thoughtfully. One of the best ways to do this is through journaling. Journaling is like a decked-out gift basket. It looks amazing. There are some delicious items on display at a glance, but it's only after you unwrap the gift that you find even more tasty treats within.

Journaling plays a prominent role in organizing your thoughts while at the same allows you the therapeutic release of bottled-up energy. If there's one special hidden gem that journaling provides is that it spotlights the beautiful synergy of order and chaos within our souls. We do a bit of a disservice by separating the two instead of accepting they are one and the same.

Once you write out your thoughts in your journal and see the words in front of you, it's real. The main critique I found that prevents some people from embracing journaling is that it comes across as a low-priority time suck. It's just another thing to do on a long list of to-dos. This is followed by a litany of grumbled excuses:

"I tried once, but I just don't have the time...", "I don't really get it. What am I supposed to write about?", etc.

None of these criticisms are wrong. I would just think of this... If journaling is simply an outlet for you to privately express yourself, free of judgment... Why wouldn't you at least take some time out of your day to journal? Don't you believe you owe it to yourself to at least try? When you take the time to explore journaling, you understand why it's so critically important to your evolution.

Here are a few pointers to get you started to gain more effective insights when you journal:

Progress: Did you accomplish your best case scenario? If yes, how does it feel? If not, why not? What can you do better next time? This is an excellent way for you to learn more about yourself and if you're in alignment with your desires, thoughts, and actions. This is where you get to be accountable for yourself.

Gratitude: Write down three things that you're grateful for. It's usually suggested 5-7. But the truth is there will be some tough days that you will struggle to reframe things. There is no perfect amount that works best for you. Just keep it real.

Check-in with your emotional state: How are you feeling now? How were you feeling most of the day? Sometimes, you're beaming with joy. Other times you're boiling over with frustration. It's easy to make note of the former but hard as hell to face the latter.

Here's the thing, when you make a note of your emotional state, it benefits you in several ways. One, you get to relieve the stress that's bothering you, even if it's for a moment, by expressing yourself openly. Two, at a later time, you will be able to check back in on your emotional state, which will give you insights into your patterns, moods, and overall well-being. This is an act of self-love. You are your best friend and your own lover. Be kind, open, and honest with yourself.

Learned Lessons: Every day there is a new lesson to learn. When you're learning, you're growing. It doesn't matter if it's big or small. Make note of it and write down what you learned. You'll thank yourself later when you look back and reflect on the critical life lessons you've accumulated over time.

Bullet Journaling: This is a popular method of personal organization developed by designer Ryder Carroll. The system organizes scheduling, reminders, to-do lists, brainstorming, and other organizational tasks into a single notebook.

Brain Dump: Brain dumping is precisely what it sounds like. It's just you dumping whatever comes to mind without judgment from your brain to paper. It can be nonsensical or incredibly thoughtful. This is an excellent technique for de-stressing. Your brain is constantly going. Whatever comes to mind, write it out, and release control. Remember, it doesn't matter how crazy it is, negative, positive, or profound. Just write it out! The goal is to simply let your random thoughts out so that your brain can take a breather.

There isn't a wrong way to journal. The real key to successful journaling is simply giving yourself the grace of time each day to journal. Do it every day. Yes, that means if you truly have nothing to say or you'd just rather not, still do it. I recommend you set aside a minimum of 15 minutes to journal twice daily. You should journal at the start of your day and at the end of your day.

When you are journaling to start your day, this is a great time to use our first core principle and to visualize how you want your day to become. You can be general, or you can be as descriptive as you wish. You should set intentions stating what you intend to accomplish through your actions. If possible, jot down your current emotional state and also the feeling you want to have if you achieve your goals for the day.

For example, it can be as simple as, *I feel like shit right now. All I want is a coffee today. Just one. I know I'll be happy the rest of the day if I have this.* Or maybe something like this, *I feel okay. Today, I want to do something selfish for myself. I'm not sure what. Maybe catch up on that show during my lunch break or end work early to catch up with a friend over drinks. That would make me feel calm.*

If nothing comes to mind. That's okay. Simply write, *This is fucking stupid. I have nothing to say.* I have found this practice to help set the day's tone. As you get into the rhythm of doing this every day, you will discover that you will have more to say than you don't.

Now, when you journal for the second time of the day, it should be more towards the end of your day. This is a great way to recap your day or even brain dump so you can rest easy. I've often jotted down my progress of the day, achievements, hard lessons learned, or even a summary. Other times I've simply written, *I'm fucking tired. Good night.* Closing your day out to a journal is not without its obstacles. There have been plenty of times after a long day at work I've found myself too exhausted to analyze anything. This is where *I'm fucking tired. Good night.* comes in handy.

Sometimes you're not alone and don't have the privacy to journal. In those cases, it's a great way to use boundaries and a healthy daily ritual to your advantage. Just simply request some time for yourself.

I discovered a new style of reflection when I wanted to develop more strategies for mental toughness. This is where I learned the technique of planning out steps for best/worst case scenarios and then outlining actionable steps I could take to get the best outcome. The deeper I went down the rabbit hole of research, I kept coming back to the training protocols of the U.S. Navy Seals. In case you didn't know, the acceptance rate of becoming a U.S. Navy Seal is astronomically low. Out of around 1,000 candidates who start the Navy Seal program each year, only about 200-250 succeed.

It's physically demanding, but even more than that, it's mentally exhausting. The whole point of their training exercises are to mentally break you to the point that you will quit. If you want to be a Seal, you have to be mentally tough. There's no way around that. If it sounds harsh, remember that the U.S. Navy Seals go on missions in maritime, jungle, urban, arctic, mountainous, and desert environments.

They are typically ordered to capture and even eliminate high-level targets or to gather intelligence behind dangerous enemy lines. This means they have to be ready for anything and everything. Their lives and the lives of countless others are determined by their choices and the speed at which they make these choices.

There is a particular training exercise that is the most difficult to pass.

It involves being underwater in a swimming pool with your scuba gear on. While you're in the pool, an instructor suddenly swims up behind you and yanks the regulator out of your mouth. You can't breathe. Then the instructor ties your oxygen lines in a knot. Holy shit. Your brain goes into survival mode. This is where the test begins.

You have to keep your cool, stay underwater, and follow procedures to get your gear back in working order so you can breathe again. This happens over and over again for 20 minutes. Only 1 out of 5 people can do this the first time. There was a commonality in a core tactic all successful candidates used to achieve success and that was... visualization.

Every day, the Seals use exercises to develop their imagery skills. With mental rehearsal, they're taught to visualize themselves succeeding in their activities and even going through the motions to achieve their ultimate goal. This outlines perfectly how you can use visualization techniques to your benefit. You jot down the problems you might encounter and simply visualize how you will overcome them.

You see, a U.S. Navy Seal spends their entire morning going over every possible mistake or potential disaster that could happen during a mission. Every possible screw-up is mercilessly examined and linked to an appropriate response: If the helicopter crash-lands, we'll do X. If we are dropped off at the wrong spot, we'll do Y. If we are outnumbered, we'll do Z. You don't have to be that extreme. You could simply jot down what you want for the day and jot down a few obstacles you could face. Again with repetition, this skill becomes stronger and stronger. This is also a fun way to explore how to overcome your daily obstacles.

I was facing a difficult obstacle of my own on a particular day and decided to use these learned reflection techniques to my advantage. The big obstacle I was facing was public speaking. A *Wall Street Journal* survey found that people ranked their number #1 fear was public speaking (even higher than being hit by a car, meaning that people would rather be run over than have to give a speech).

My speech had high stakes. I had a very important presentation to provide to my client, an impulsive but charming CEO of a tech startup and his core technical team.

He even flew me out from Los Angeles, California to Austin Texas for this presentation. As a Marketing Consultant, the task was simple enough. I just needed to best explain how to best market his product and what the future outlook could look like with me leading the initiatives. So, in the morning, I started my day journaling. Then I used visualization techniques to map out my day.

First, the best-case scenario. Then three to four steps I could take to make sure the best-case scenario would happen for me. Then I took a look at the worst-case scenario: *What if everything was a disaster that day?* The best case scenario is that I would go into the presentation, armed with enough knowledge in my tactics that I could answer any question thrown at me. I needed to know my game plan in and out.

I wanted to be fresh, well-groomed, and energetic. My presentation would go over so well, that not only would I wow everyone in the room but, the CEO would be impressed enough to give me a bonus and extend our contract. I'd play it cool and accept the amazing response. Then I wrote down the worst-case scenario. I'd show up late.

I wouldn't be able to play my presentation properly. When it was time to give it, I'd fumble my words. That would only make me even more nervous and I would completely forget everything I knew. I'd be buzzing with too much adrenaline to have a focused thought. Everyone would notice.

The CEO would walk out of the room embarrassed. The rest of the team would snicker under their breaths or even worse, just stare ahead with a deafening silence. So, I thought it over for a few minutes. Then I wrote easy actionable steps I could take to get the outcome I wanted:

1. Craft a presentation that summarizes my game plan.
2. Practice my presentation in front of the mirror.
3. Go to the meeting location early. Walk around to get out any last minute jitters.
4. Stick to what you know.

When the time came for my presentation, I got there early just as I had planned. But, the CEO and his team were already there. Once the CEO saw me, he rushed to me, filling me in with the latest developments with a hushed whisper. He informed me that one of his key investors flew in to attend the presentation personally. Not just the investor came either, but also team-members of an outside (and local) PR firm that he had also hired was also going to be attending as well. Now, I should mention that this particular PR firm was more than just a bit interested to see what marketing strategy I had in mind, most importantly what role they would play in it.

This didn't throw me off my game though. This wasn't even something I planned for even in my worst case scenario. When it came to my actual presentation, there were indeed technical issues, but I resolved them quickly. I gave a riveting presentation. I was calm, energetic, but most of all I was well-informed. Eyes were glued to the visuals of my presentation. Everyone was leaning forward, locked in. By the end, there were no questions. Just an energetic applause. Everyone was pleased and the CEO did extend my contract (no raise or bonus though).

Now, even though I used an example from a page out of my professional life, you'll notice that my fears were all personal and tied to my own identity and insecurities. As I stated before, your personal and professional lives work in tandem. If I'm being mindful of my state of well-being then that will ultimately have an impression on my work abilities. I focused on what I could control and understood there were things that could potentially happen out of my control. So, I did what I could to minimize the negative outcomes. I let go of the ones I couldn't.

Visualization gives us an opportunity to focus on what we desire first. Secondly, it gives us the chance to tackle our fears head-on, organize the steps we need to take to achieve what we want, and ultimately present our goals as attainable. Now, let's apply the power of visualization to help us understand the type of action we need to take in our lives.

Imagine if it's next Tuesday and you had everything you ever wanted. What would your life be like from the moment you woke up to the moment you went to sleep? Answer this question for yourself in writing. When you do this, try to be as detailed as you can. From the feelings, you have throughout your perfect day to the people you encounter (or even don't).

Just use your imagination and let your desires flow from pen to paper. No judgment. No problem-solving. Just be honest with yourself about what your perfect day looks like. After working out this particular visualization exercise, I have discovered people slip into three groups.

The first group of people doesn't even bother performing the exercise. They use the excuse of not having enough time or the inability to think of anything to jot down. If you fall into this category, be sure to look back at the lessons learned in our first two principles. This will allow you to break down what's holding you back from simply imagining what your perfect day would look like.

The second group tends to be brief about what their day is like. Usually, this is a combination of work tasks, hobbies, and spending quality time with loved ones. Other times it's a day off on a dream vacation or winning the lottery. One visualization someone shared with me looked like this, "I walk my dog and get coffee. Then I went to work. No one bothered me. It was great. After work, I hang out with my friends. I get really drunk and take a beautiful girl home with me. We have a night of wild sex. We smoke and talk about life in bed for a while. That's about it."

The final group of people go all the way in. These are the ones that are so descriptive that it's abundantly clear that they know exactly what they want and how they want it. Some are incredibly grounded and logical. Some are very imaginative. But, in both cases, they're very detailed and clearly depict what a perfect day would look like for them.

One glowing example from the third group is a very successful friend of mine who, at the time, was a fellow skilled photographer and is now an entrepreneur. At the time, she was single and frustrated with the lack of commitment and follow-through from romantic relationships. Even though she had a thriving business, she mainly worked alone and was getting burnt out from working all the time. When I asked her to do this visualization exercise, she had a detailed response ready to go. She was one of the more vivid and detailed storytellers I've come across.

She told me, "I woke up with my dog licking my face. The sun's coming up, and we go for a walk on the beach to catch the sunrise. I don't wake up early right now, but I'd like to start. After we get settled in, I make some breakfast. I imagine that my friends would come over and join me for breakfast."

She beamed with excitement as she continued, "We will talk about life, work, and the troubles that we face in life. Afterward, I would go on a production set. I'm not as hands-on as I am right now. I have a team that has everything set up for me. In fact, I just want to stroll onto the set and just focus on my subject. I wouldn't mind doing one or two production shoots a day. Right now, I do three to five and have to wrangle everything. I don't want to do that anymore. After work, I'd go to dinner with my boyfriend."

She's really energized now. She isn't just answering a question, she's *living* in this moment., "We're having a lovely dinner near the beach or watching the sunset. It's very romantic. We can talk about anything. We go back to my place, and we dance to music. There's a lot of laughter in our home. We enjoy each other's company. We make love. We sleep in each other's arms. My dog is lying at the foot of the bed. It's all very sweet, calm, and romantic."

After my friend shared her visualization with me, I followed up with her routinely to ask if she had made any progress. Every time she gave me an update, there was something new. She was taking small steps. First inward. Then outward. Professionally and personally, in tandem.

Before long, she realized her perfect day. Just the way she imagined it. Full of love, success, and happiness. When I followed up with the first group, I discovered the opposite result. Most of them still didn't perform the "perfect day" exercise for a variety of different reasons. Some said it made them feel bad because it seemed too unattainable. Others didn't really get the point of doing the exercise in the first place. Everyone promised they would get around to trying the exercise… "one day".

I received mixed responses from the second group. It was either a work in progress, or they forgot about doing the exercise entirely. Everyone from the third group, including my friend, found consistency in the progress they were making. So, what gives? Why did my friend and others like her reach her perfect day?

The answer is hidden in the details. This last group used the "perfect day" exercise to have a clear understanding of what they wanted. Even more than that, they had a blueprint that they could make a game plan from. They understood that details matter. They further understood that just by clearly seeing what they wanted to excite them.

They were of an abundance mindset to harness the power of reflection and visualization. They understand that they're the group of people that don't ask, "What is the worst that can happen?" but instead a question we should all be asking ourselves, "What's the best that can happen?"

CHAPTER EIGHT

The Discovery of Self

The discovery of self is critical to your journey of empowerment and growth. This is directly tied to reflection. The definition of self-reflection is the exercising of introspection, coupled with the willingness to learn about yourself, in order to help you achieve self-awareness. By becoming more self-aware, you are able to better control how you react to things and how to focus your attention to the most beneficial areas of your life. When you take the time to become more self-aware, you'll discover several truths about yourself and the world around you.

Things are never as bad as you think they are. You're more powerful than you always thought. You are not the center of the universe, and there isn't anything wrong with that. Your feelings should be respected, but they should not dominate your decision making. The history of you is done and over with. What truly matters is who you are now and who you ultimately want to become.

You can do this by exploring your core values, principles, and boundaries. Now, we can explore how you can use them to your advantage to find more self-awareness. Understanding who you are at your core isn't just a way to annihilate the false narratives that we created for ourselves. It also allows us to embrace the growing pains of life while gaining perspective.

Let's try the following exercise to see how well you know yourself by exploring your own core values, principles, and boundaries. Understanding which means the most to you will have you in alignment with your integrity. This will make it easier to take on life's obstacles and live a more fulfilled life. For this exercise, I want you to look inwards and take these steps discover your most important core values:

1. First, list out your top 10 core values. When you craft your list be sure to rank your values on a scale from 1-10, putting the ones you identify with and the most important to you at the top of your list.

2. Next, let's narrow down your list and focus on the top three values you feel define the best version of yourself. This will allow you to understand more about what truly makes you tick.

3. Pay close attention to your top core value that means the most to you. When you know what this is, use it as your guiding north star. Your anchor for stability. When the world throws out its inevitable challenges, use your values as a way to respond to anything thrown at you. For example, if *loyalty* is the value you care the most about then you should explore how you're loyal to yourself and others. Maybe you're not feeling devoted to achieving your own goals, or perhaps you feel like you're doing a great job being loyal to your family.

One may be something that needs improvement, and the latter is something that makes you proud. Either way, it goes, you're making progress by just exploring your values.

4. Next, let's make note of your top five principles. You'll discover principles that take a little more time to explore.

5. Once you have our top five principles down, trim it down to your top three. These are the leading principles you want to live by. For example, a principle I have listed for myself is that I would like to see inconveniences as lessons to be learned and opportunities for growth.

6. Finally, write down ten of your non-negotiable boundaries. This is a list of deal-breakers that you must enforce with yourself, family, friends, romantic partners, co-workers, etc. This list of boundaries is where you draw a line in the sand about what you deem acceptable and not acceptable for yourself. For example, you might have to stick to your budget as your most crucial boundary. You might notice that you'd like to show respect for differences in opinion, perspective, and feelings when you chat with someone with opposing views. We're going to continue with our rule of threes and choose your top three boundaries.

7. We're going to continue with our rule of threes and choose your top three boundaries. Once you've completed this final task you will have a polished list of the values, principles, and boundaries that mean the most to you.

The above exercise is a great practice for understanding who you are as a person. I want you to carry your values, principles, and boundaries with you at all times. You can reference them on those tough days or confusing times of your life. You should continuously update these lists as you change and grow. You'll discover that some things don't carry the same impact they once did. That's a good sign that you're continuously evolving.

When we discuss ways to create more opportunities for reflection, we can't leave out the art of mediation. The two are intertwined because meditation is a great tool for self-awareness. Meditation is a set of techniques that are intended to encourage a heightened state of awareness and focused attention. When implemented correctly, meditation can serve as a great tool for life and mood improvement. The reason why meditation is so powerful is that it causes shifts in our awareness. We tend to over-identify with our thoughts and emotions, which can prolong them and make them feel bigger than they are, especially the ones that impact us negatively.

Those types of thoughts or feelings can agonize us for days on end. Meditation provides you with a sense of calm, peace and balance that can benefit both your emotional well-being and your overall health. You can also use it to relax and cope with stress by refocusing your attention on something calming. Meditation can help you learn to stay centered and keep inner peace.

Reflection gives us insight into our own thoughts. It allows us to understand how we operate and gives us insight into our strengths and weaknesses. With practicing meditation you can receive extraordinary results like improving your working memory and fluid intelligence, allowing the space for better stress management skills and critical thinking, improving your emotional well-being, and provide you a better management of symptoms of health conditions including anxiety disorders, depression, sleep disorders, pain issues, and high blood pressure.

While it's abundantly clear that there are so many benefits from meditating, the real struggle for so many of us is making time to do it in the first place. There were times in my life when I was so busy with my work that I woke up, got ready for work, commuted to work, worked my ass off, ate at my desk, worked more, and then went home. I was so exhausted from the day that I just vegged out in front of my TV. Small talk with a loved one. Then I'm too tired to do anything.

Can you relate? How in the hell would I have time to meditate? Or maybe you *do* have the time but don't have the space for it? Or perhaps you have a clingy friend, noisy roommates, a hovering girlfriend, loud-ass neighbors, or a constant barrage of phone notifications. Perhaps meditating just isn't your thing, so you have zero desire to do it.

It's funny how we create more excuses not to do something that benefits us than find opportunities to do it. How odd is that? Let's try this on for size. We have already explored ways to look within ourselves and face challenges head-on. Could you take on the challenge of finding 5-10 minutes a day for yourself to meditate?

Don't think about meditation as another obligation, do it because it's a great expression of loving yourself. I like meditating in the mornings as a part of my routine. Meditating in the morning is a lot like washing your face. Just like you wash your face to feel clean, rejuvenated, and ready for the day, taking out time to breathe first thing upon awakening does wonders for you. Meditating in the morning clears away residual tension from your dreams or nightmares, self-limiting beliefs, and even anxious thoughts about the day ahead. If you can't find time to do it in the mornings, meditate during your natural gaps between your daily activities.

Like after you get ready and before you head out the door, between tasks at work, after cooking and before you start to eat. As often as you can, use these transition times to close your eyes and take 3-5 natural, relaxed breaths. Even just a minute or so of conscious breathing and stillness helps de-escalate your stress response and brings you back to your center. You can do this anywhere (at your desk, in your car, in the bathroom, at home), sitting or standing with a tall spine. The more you practice taking very brief meditation breaks, the more it becomes your natural response to turn to your breath in stressful situations.

When you do make the time to meditate be sure to just… breathe. Breathing plays a critical role in mediation. Breathe naturally and notice the feelings and sensations that you experience as you breathe in and out. Don't try to suppress your feelings. Your mind is bound to wander as you meditate.

Sometimes this can lead to thoughts and feelings that are uncomfortable or even distressing. The goal isn't to clear your mind of such ideas. This is one of the biggest misconceptions about meditation. Most people that don't practice meditation enough or know enough about it think you can just shut off your brain, and that's the end of it.

No, of course not. Instead, acknowledge these thoughts without judging them, and then gently guide your focus back toward your breathing. Breathing is always your point of focus in all forms of meditation.

After you put in the work of reflection, it can be both exhilarating and draining at first. It's okay to get your mind onto something else afterward just to decompress. Whether that be taking your mind off things by playing video games, catching up on a movie or your favorite tv shows, spending time with your friends and family, or even meditating more. You will notice that the world will feel quite different from what it did before. You will be more enlightened now. You will feel much better about things, about your lifestyle, about yourself, and that's the whole point.

Just like I said before, putting the practice of reflection into your life can be difficult. When I began my journey into photography, my subject was one of my best friends, Mikey. I've known him since I was in college and got to witness first-hand how he evolved over the years. If you were to look at my portfolio at the early stages of my creative career, you would see his bearded face on almost everything. At this stage of his life, he was a bearded hipster who was getting restless at being stuck in a cubicle at his 9 to 5 job. Soon he would explore more of his creative passions just as much as I was.

Mikey was adaptable to any art form, whether it be acting, music, or photography. He's the type of person that often laughs (even at himself). His infectious laugh would have you doubled over in giggling fits with him. Like all of us, Mikey was exploring more about life, who he was, and where he was going. He eventually joined our group of buddies on challenging hikes. It became more prevalent in Mikey's lifestyle and the new identity he was forming for himself.

Around that same time, it was the beginning stages of a chaotic chapter of my life that I mentioned before in this book. So, outside of periodic hangout sessions and photoshoots, I was wrapped up in my own world. As time passed, I had less time for our friendship. That's how it goes sometimes, isn't it?

One morning I was rushing out of a meeting with a client when a friend kept buzzing me. When I finally answered, his voice was quaking with pain. He simply said, "Mikey's *gone*." My senses froze when I heard those two words. My friends and I pull pranks on each other all the time. Was this one of them, I thought to myself? The way in which my friend uttered those words, though, and just the time of his call… I understood it was real.

As it turned out, the night before, Michael went on a date with a girl he met on a dating app. To impress her, he took her out on a hike on Mt. Whitney. I know this to be true because we texted the night before he went on his date. It was our last text together. Me wishing him luck on his date. He and his date went on their hike around 7:30 pm.

While hiking down the trail, they got lost and separated. He was heard falling along with the sound of tumbling rocks. His date made her way back to the Outpost camp to get help. They would eventually find his body in a chute near Mirror Lake. It took me a long time to process all of my feelings about all of it.

At times, I was angry with him for being so reckless. Other times, I would be struck with guilt for being angry with him. But mostly, I was just sad that he was gone. It did feel like a piece of me was forever gone. At one point, I made an unconscious decision to push my grief so deep down inside that any memories and relationships that included him became fuzzy and distant.

This even includes pushing away my group of friends. I would ask the wrong questions, mulling over what I could have done to be a better friend or even intervene to prevent him from going on a hiking date in the first place. Even worse, I would mull over what his final moments were like, and how scared he must have felt. These types of thoughts and questions would keep me up most nights, pondering even my own mortality. I would avoid any sort of healthy reflection.

Instead I would try to avoid any memories of our bond and friendship altogether. After his death, I went through a lot of low points in my career and personal life that I shared with you. This, however, was the one thing I always had trouble facing. I honestly don't know why. Grieving someone you care about is difficult. For each one of us, we have our own way of dealing with it, and it's impossible to predict how you will act or feel in this kind of situation.

Eventually, through the help of therapy and the exercises I mentioned earlier, I mourned my lost friend. I had to accept the reality of what had happened and how much my good friend meant to me. I started asking the right questions that led to me accepting what had happened and continuing to keep his memory alive in the creative pursuits I took. I would eventually reflect on our friendship through journaling, meditating, and even therapy. It was tough to sharpen my focus on the very things I tried so hard to push out of my mind for so long after his sudden death.

I understood however that I needed to confront what I was avoiding for so long to finally heal from the pain I felt from losing my friend. There was one great lesson that I took from our friendship that I will share with you. That is the lesson of not taking your life or anyone that you care about for granted. If it hasn't become abundantly clear yet, your life is what you make of it. Cherish the small moments just as much as you do the big ones.

Take nothing for granted because nothing is guaranteed. Nothing is owed to us even though we'd like to pretend it is. It's truly not. If you want something, you'll have to get it yourself. If you care about someone, don't assume they know.

Tell them. This is your moment. Right now. Don't let it slip away.

ACTIONS

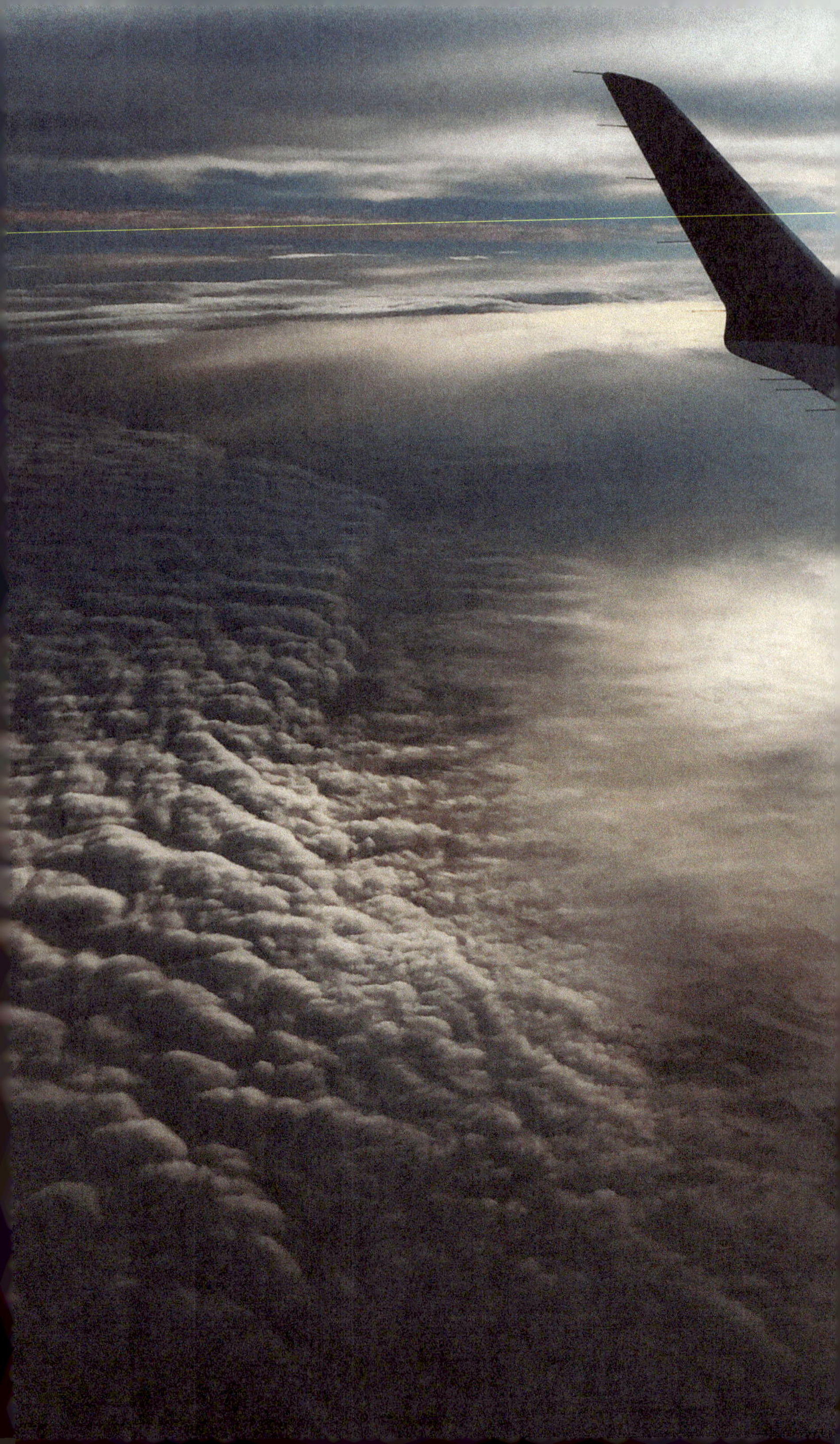

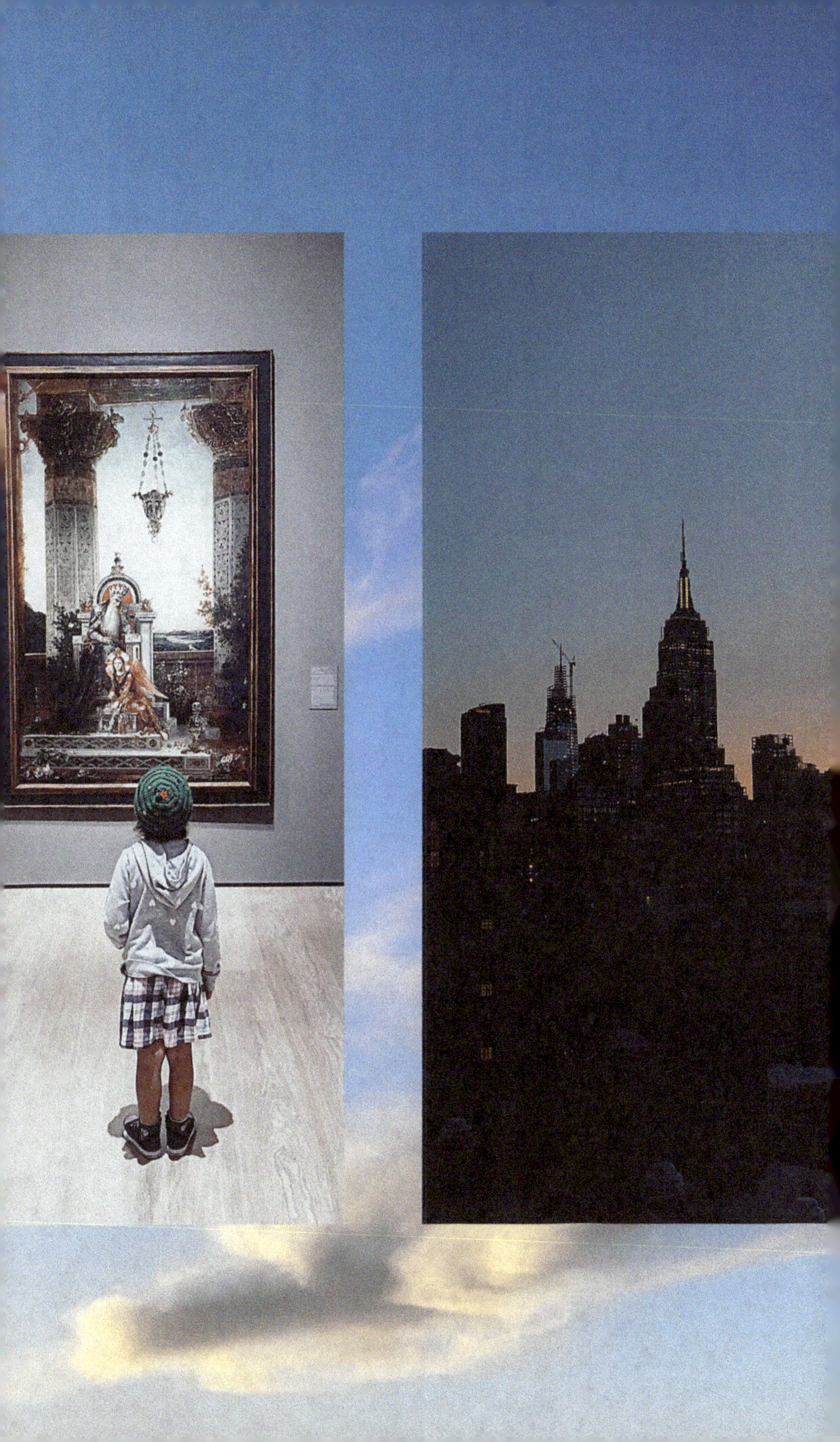

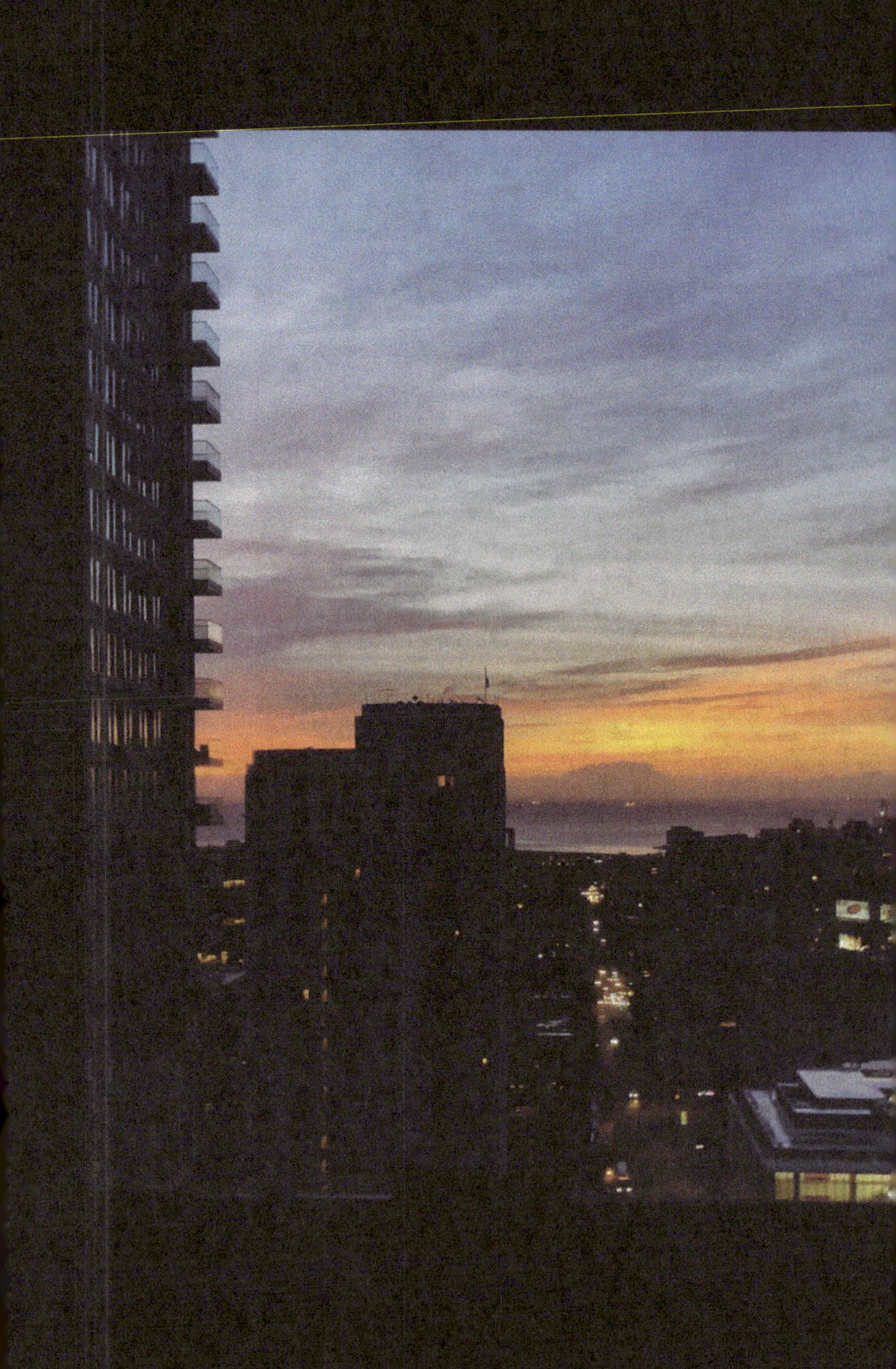

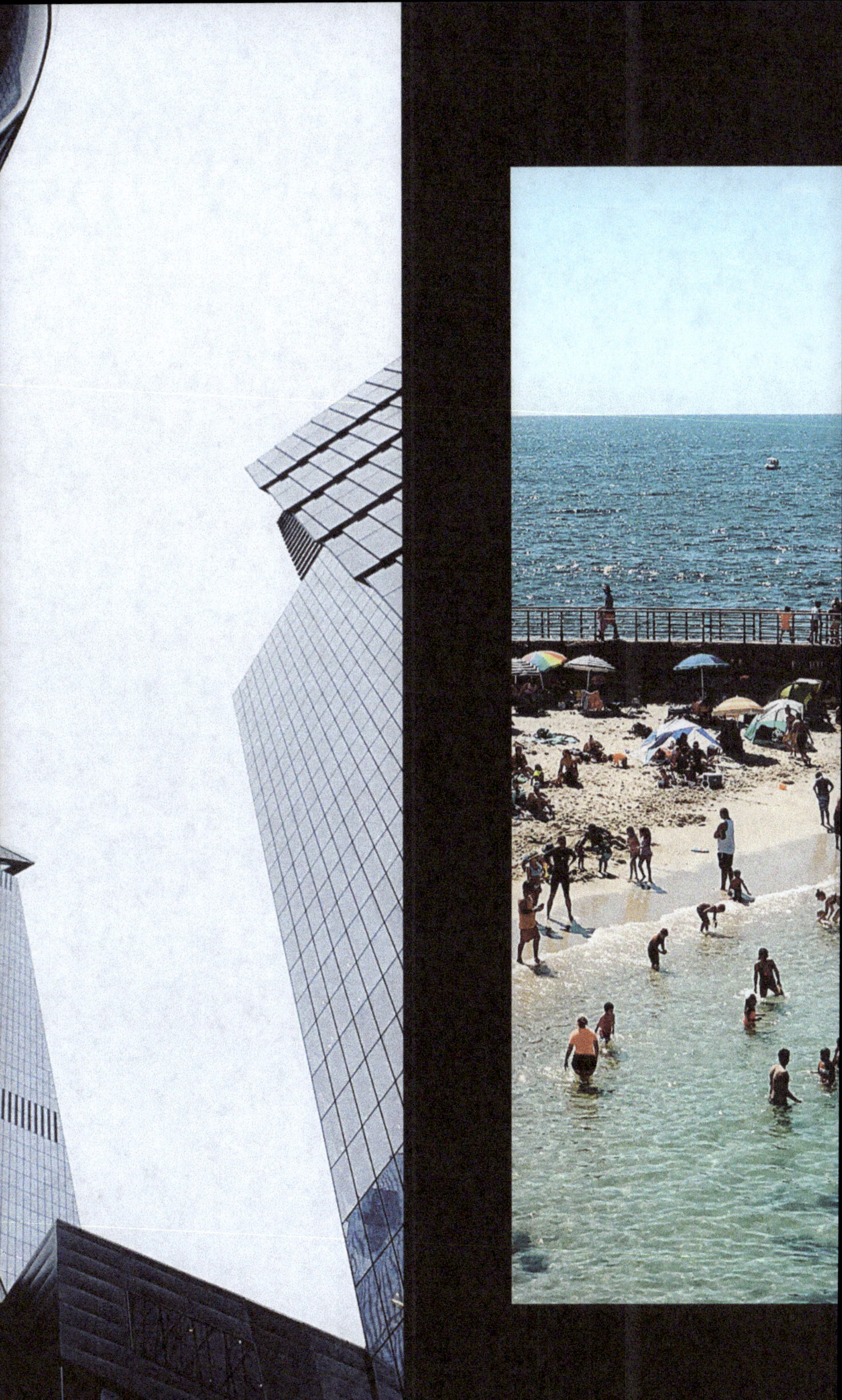

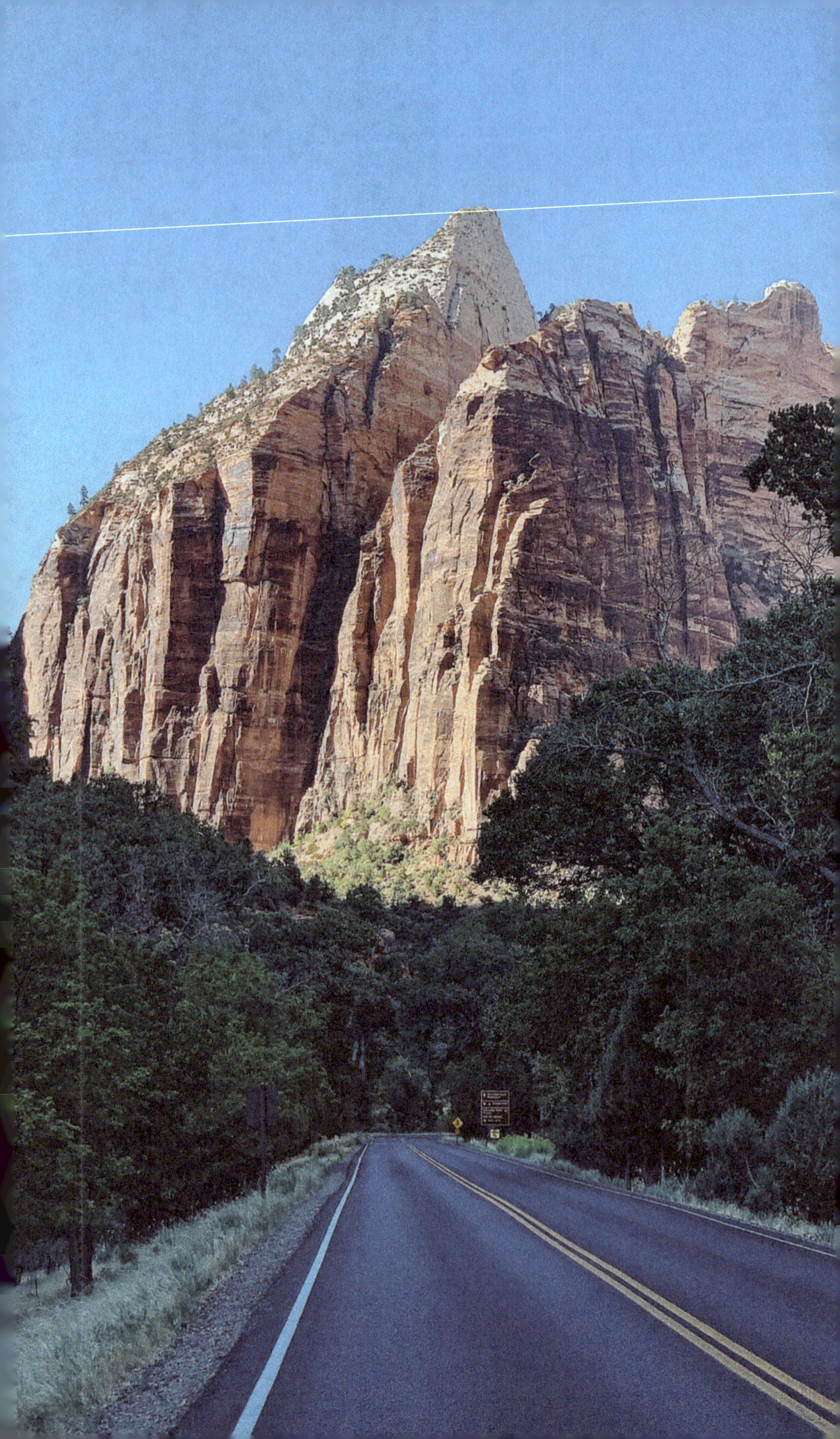

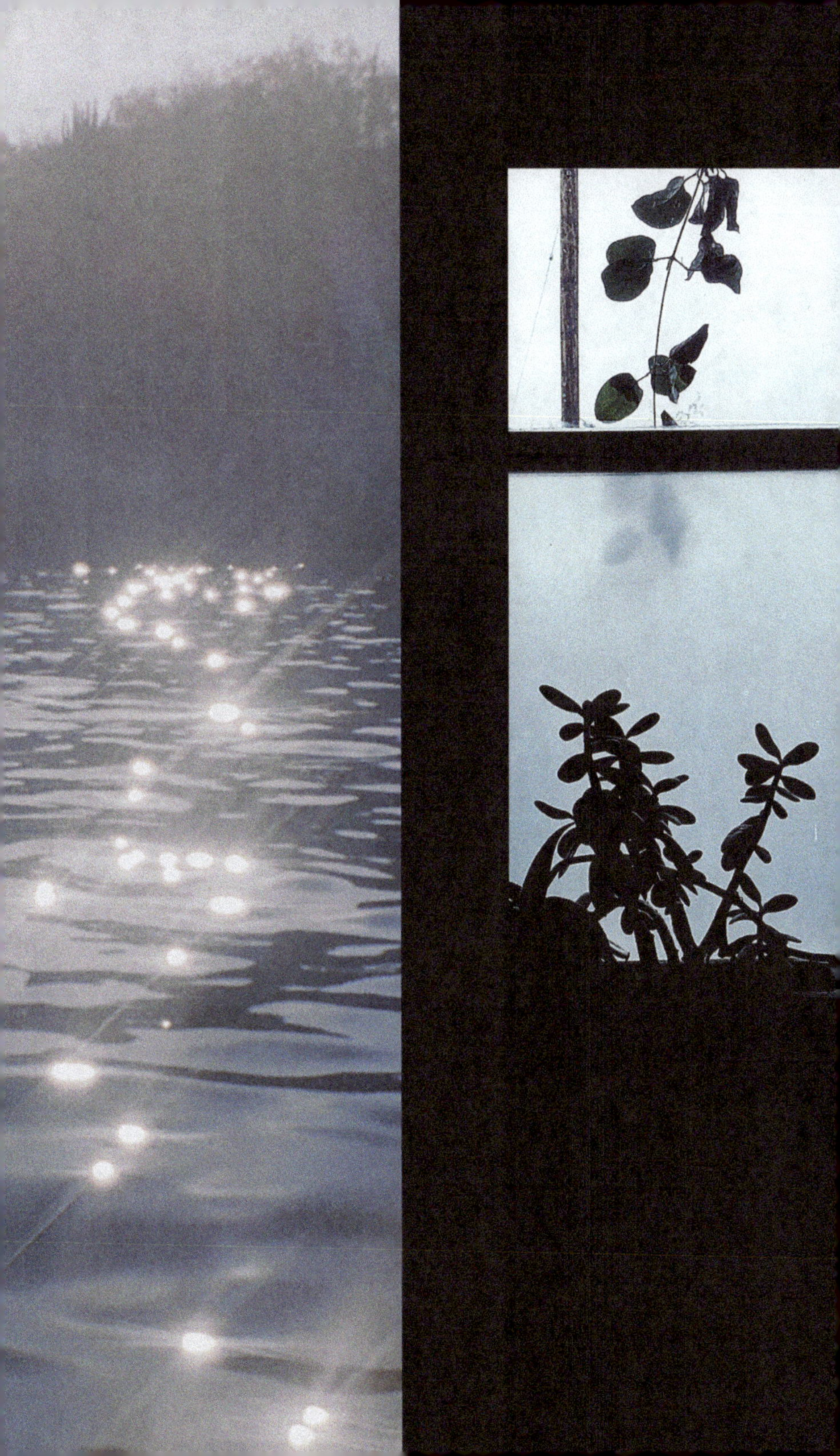

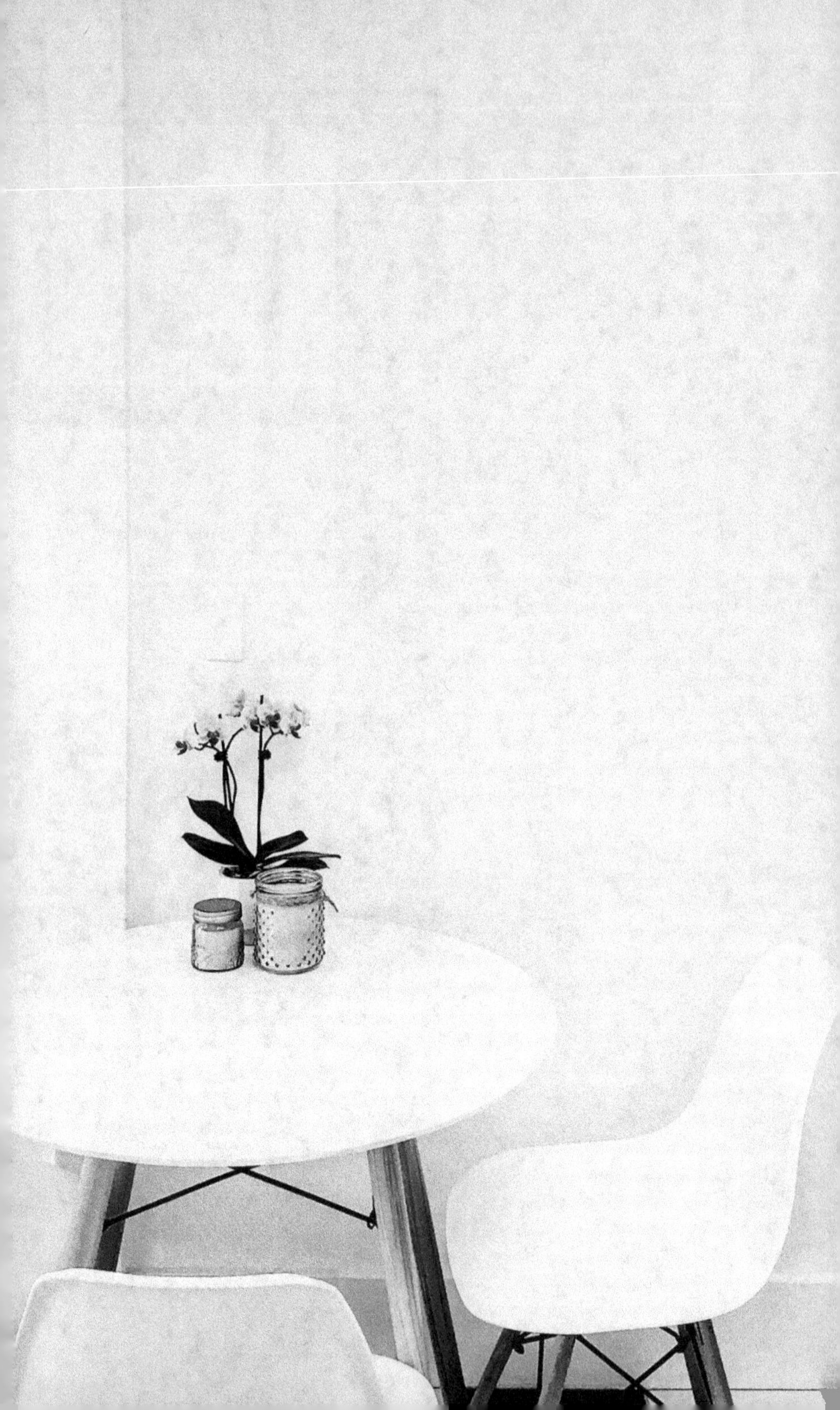

CHAPTER NINE

The Fear Factor

We learned to ask better questions. Armed with the ability to ask the right questions, we can find a clearer path to achieving our desires and goals. When we reflect, we're achieving a heightened state of self-awareness that can turn our pain into power. We can understand our motivations and the steps we need to take to get what we want. It only makes sense that what comes next is to take bold *action*.

In this section, we'll discuss how to put those questions and reflections in motion to obtain your desired outcome. Bold action is what will transform our lives. Remember that if your intention is powerful, your actions will also be powerful. If your actions are powerful, then you will always achieve something special for yourself and the people around you. With this principle of action, we will explore how taking even small incremental steps can lead to more significant outcomes.

Often, we know what we need to do, but we get stuck on *how* to do it. Even more than that, the *why*. This is why our first two principles are so critical to do before you take a course of action. We need to be clear on our motivations first. I could easily say, "Hey, if you want to book a ticket to Bali for the first time, go book that one-way ticket now! Worry about the rest later!"

It's true that impulsive action removes the fear and overthinking factors quickly. A great example of using impulsive action to your advantage is *The 5 Second Rule* principle, created by author Mel Robbins. The principle is that if you have an instinct to act on a goal, you must physically move within 5 seconds to achieve this goal, or your brain will kill it. That principle does work, just not for everyone. Some actions are much more strategic.

The ones where you are laying out steps of action with a lot of thought. The truth is, you must create the ability to adapt to any situation, so you instinctively know the best course of action. Your dreams become a reality when you put an idea into action. The more intentional action you take the more opportunities you'll create to get what you want. There will always be obstacles that will prevent you from acting.

We'll be in excellent shape if we learn what they are and how to face them head-on. I have found there to be three major challenges that prevent us from taking action: fear, confusion, and burnout. We will explore all three within the principle of action and how you can overcome them. You must first understand why it's so difficult for you to take action and how you can overcome those obstacles. This won't just increase your chances of finding (and maintaining) the success and happiness that you're looking for, but it will also save you time.

There is nothing more mystifying and challenging to your own progress than fear. Fear is the ultimate challenge to overcome. No one is immune to fear. It can seize control of our lives and send us down the road of unfulfilled destinies. That's a great tragedy. Fear comes in many forms. There are five basic fears, out of which almost all of our other so-called fears are manufactured. These fears include extinction, mutilation, loss of autonomy, separation, and ego death (as we learned earlier in this book). The universal trigger for fear is the threat of harm, real or imagined. This threat can be against our physical, emotional or psychological well-being. While there are certain things that trigger fear in most of us, we can learn to become afraid of nearly anything. Fear itself causes hesitation, poor judgment, lack of confidence, and endings before actual beginnings. Personally, professionally, it doesn't matter. Fear cripples you into inaction.

Imagine a scenario where you enjoy your job, know the value you bring to the table and want a promotion. Yet you don't know how you should ask about it. You don't even know where to start. So, you overthink it, and then you wait… and wait… and wait… until you decide to… delay your ask. Instead of doing anything about it, you seek out advice.

Then you think about it some more. At that stage, you've blown past a healthy reflection stage or didn't even act swiftly on the advice you sought out. In fact, you blew past the very thing you knew to be true at the beginning, which is that you bring value. You want something in return that you think you rightfully deserve. Simple.

Maybe you need to have a much needed conversation with someone you're afraid to have. Perhaps you're afraid to chase after your true dreams and passions. Instead of choosing to let fear take control of your life, let's face it head on. We can do this by simply applying the principles of *The Maguire Method*.

Let's make our fears less complex and empower yourself to not get in your own way. Remember that the self is the root of all fear. To inhibit or suppress fear is not to transcend it. Instead through the discovery of self it can be understood and dissolved. First, ask yourself the good types of questions that help you not just confront your own fears but minimize their impact. Here are 24 questions you should be asking yourself:

1. What is the worst thing that can happen if I go after my goals?
2. What is the best thing that can happen if I go after my goals?
3. Is it worth it to go all in?
4. What am I *actually* afraid of?
5. Am I afraid of the process or the result?
6. Do I feel that I can handle the process?
7. Do I feel like I can handle the outcome?
8. Do I feel confident in my abilities to perform?
9. Do I feel that I must perform but I really don't want to?
10. Am I pressuring myself to make a decision quickly when I don't have enough information?
11. What is the information that I need exactly to feel ready?
12. Am I trying to protect myself from a particular outcome? If so, why?
13. Can I read a book, take a class, do more research to feel more knowledgeable?
14. Do I know someone who has been in this position before who can provide details around what currently feels abstract and scary?
15. Would I be willing to ask that someone honest questions?
16. Am I scared that I may make a mistake?
17. Am I allowed to make mistakes?
18. Am I scared of being wrong?
19. Is my self-worth tied to being right? If so, why?
20. Can I allow myself to be wrong?

21. Can I allow myself to feel an overwhelming feeling and know that it will pass?
22. If a person has a negative opinion of me, what impact will that have to my day-to-day life?
23. When was the last time I felt this fear?
24. Will I be able to handle this situation differently than the last time I felt this specific fear?

Next, reflect on the answers you discover for yourself when you ask these questions about fear. Analyze your responses. Think about how they made you feel. Visualize a game plan for yourself. Then take swift action for yourself.

If you want that promotion and you think you deserve it, simply lay out the reasons why, and explain to your supervisor or boss those reasons. It would be a smart move to further explain what other intangibles you can bring to your job upon promotion. Every situation is different in how you can do this, but the key here is to take swift action for yourself.

Don't let fear stop you. Maybe there's somebody that you've met in your life that when you're with that person, it makes you feel at home. You've been dating for some time and want to make it official. You just don't know how to navigate that conversation out of fear of rejection. So… you say nothing at all. When in reality, you could have just been open and honest early on so you could put your mind at ease. Even if you didn't get what you wanted, you didn't have to waste more time on something that didn't match up to the reality of what you wanted.

Do not focus on what happens if you fail. Instead, ask a better question. What if, instead, you asked yourself what is there to be gained? What if you asked for that promotion, and you got it just like you asked for? What if you did have that conversation with someone that you really like, and it turns out that they feel the same way and even more over the moon about you than you are about them? We have already learned how to ask better questions and reflect in a healthy way to get more clarity on the necessary steps to take. Don't let the fear stop you.

One type of fear that sneaks up on us is the fear of failure. The underlying cause of the fear of failure is actually fear of shame or embarrassment. The actual incident, like failing a test, not winning that race, or not finishing that book you swore you'd write. It's the accompanying emotion of worthlessness that it provokes. Understand this. Failure is unavoidable. You will fail. That is one of the certainties of life.

You win some, and you lose some. Sometimes it will be embarrassing for everyone to see. Other times it will be private. Either way, failure in life is inevitable. It's so unavoidable that it's pretty humorous when you think about how scared we can be about making decisions that will bring us more satisfaction just out of fear of failing. Why are you so frightened of taking the action that will get you what you want most out of your life?

Nearly all of the inspiring success stories come from epic failures, like a bizarrely outrageous idea from Gary Dahl. In 1975, Gary Dahl was an advertising executive with a crazy idea. Gary believed consumers would pay good money for a more convenient pet than a dog or a cat… your very own pet rock. Obviously, the idea sounded bizarre, and not a single bank would lend him a dime to start marketing such a goofy product. Did Dahl sink back in embarrassment and back off?

No. He doubled down on his idea and even took out a second mortgage on his house. He invested in advertising his product in magazines and newspapers. Just as everyone had predicted, the pet rock was a colossal failure. Dahl didn't see it that way, though. With his last $200, Dahl placed a small ad in a Chicago newspaper, marketing his pet rock as an ideal Christmas present.

The plan worked this time around. Enough people were amused by the idea of giving a piece of granite for the holidays. In all, Dahl sold over 1.5 million rocks for $3.95 for each product. Obviously, the fad didn't last long, but it didn't need to. Dahl became a millionaire off of the idea of owning your very own pet rock. Dahl proves that even the strangest ideas that fail repeatedly are still worth exploring.

We also have the opportunity to become our best selves through failure and reveal our steadfast perseverance, like in the story of Jack Andraka. When Jack was 15, he wanted to create a diagnostic test for pancreatic cancer that was better than the tests developed by scientists, research labs, and billion-dollar pharmaceutical companies. Jack wrote a proposal to develop a better test. 199 research labs rejected him. However, the 200th research lab, Johns Hopkins University in Baltimore, Maryland, said, "Yes." At the lab, Jack Andraka developed a pancreatic cancer test that was 100 times better and 26,000 times less expensive than the current test. Jack's invention will save tens of thousands of lives.

Then there is the story of Nick Woodman, who had his own embarrassing public failure. Nick Woodman's startup, Funbug, was backed with $3.9 million from investors. Funbug failed with $3.9 million down the drain. Woodman was so devastated that he took an extended surfing trip. Woodman wanted to take videos while he was surfing. That led to his next idea.

What if people had cameras that made it easy for them to video record while participating in activities? Woodman and his girlfriend sold shell necklaces out of the trunk of their car to raise money for his idea. They also borrowed money from Woodman's parents. In 2002, Woodman launched GoPro, and by 2014, he became a billionaire. Nick Woodman would eventually lose his billionaire title but still remain a multimillionaire and successful entrepreneur.

It's hard to believe that one of the most recognizable names in online publications, Arianna Huffington, was once rejected by three dozen major publishers. Huffington's second book, which she tried to publish long before she created the now ubiquitously recognizable *Huffington Post* empire, was rejected 36 times before it was eventually accepted for publication. Even *Huffington Post* itself wasn't a success right away. In fact, when it launched, there were dozens of highly negative reviews about its quality and its potential. Obviously, Huffington overcame those initial bouts of failure and has cemented her name as one of the most successful outlets on the web.

Then there are the private failures that lead to game-changing triumphs. Due to sexism, Elizabeth Blackwell was rejected from 29 medical schools. So, she went to visit the schools in person. She was told she should pretend to be a man because women weren't fit to receive medical schooling. She refused.

Blackwell was accepted by mistake by Hobart College (then Geneva Medical College), and she enrolled. Many doctors refused to work with her, but she persevered and eventually graduated. Elizabeth Blackwell became the first woman to receive a medical degree in the United States in 1849. She then built her own medical practice, created a place where women could have medical internships (since many healthcare facilities didn't welcome women), served impoverished families, and established the first medical university for women.

Like I said before, we will all fail. So, what's the point of fearing that you will? You take a leap of faith to follow your own path instead of the one you think you're supposed to walk. You never know what that will lead to.

Vera Wang's early career started out like many others. She worked a full-time job at someone else's company. She spent 15 years working her way up at *Vogue*. However, after repeatedly getting rejected for the Editor in Chief position, she realized that her career at *Vogue* just wouldn't go any further. This led to her becoming a fashion designer and building a name for herself in the wedding gown industry. Today, Vera Wang's dresses have been worn by countless celebrities, and her company makes more than $343.8 million in revenue each year, employing nearly 200 people. Her net worth is estimated to be $420 million.

Famous failures like Vera Wang's teach you two core lessons. First, you can build up a wealth of knowledge while working a 9 to 5 job that you can apply to your future business (if that's something you want). Secondly, she's a great example of knowing when to adapt and pivot. By realizing she wasn't going to get the Editor in Chief role, she opened up the possibility of taking on an opportunity much more incredible than Vogue could ever offer.

According to a New York Times piece, Dr. Kerry Ressler, Director of the Neurobiology of Fear Laboratory at McLean Hospital, stated, "Fear is the most evolutionarily conserved behavioral reflex for survival." He further added that 10% of people generalize fearful memories or grief. Their brains continually get cues that bad things are still happening, and their bodies respond accordingly. 90% are resilient after something frightening or tragic happens, like a car accident or the death of a loved one. They are left with a bad memory or with grief, but they have a new perspective.

It doesn't matter where you came from. It only matters where you're going. There are always lessons to be learned in failure. Instead of seeing failures as something personal against you, see them instead as a better roadmap in how you need to sharpen your vision, an opportunity to grow, and understand the lesson you need to learn.

CHAPTER TEN

Too Much of a Good Thing

In too many instances, we have so many notifications, choices, and polarizing opinions that by the time we are alone with our thoughts and unplug, some of us are left completely drained. It's not just the number of choices we have at our disposal but the polarization of our choices. Countless studies and research have consistently held that people with fewer options tend to make better and easier decisions than those with too many. When did having too many choices become too good of a thing?

According to the book *The Paradox of Choice* written by Psychologist and Professor of Social Theory Barry Schwartz, "If we're rational, social scientists tell us, added options can only make us better off as a society. This view is logically compelling, but empirically it isn't true." As it turns out, having too many options is particularly confounding when the information available on them is limited or confusing.

Consumer behavioral studies help us understand more about this. Many brands and retailers now wield marketing buzzwords such as "curation", "differentiation", and "discovery" as they attempt to sell an assortment of stuff targeted to their ideal customer.

Companies find such shoppers through the data gold mine of digital advertising, which can catalog people by gender, income level, personal interests, and more. We have truly lost the ability to sort through the sheer volume of the consumer choices available to us. A ghost now has to be in the retail machine, whether it's an algorithm, an influencer, or some snazzy ad technology to help a product follow you around the internet.

Choice fatigue is one of the very reasons why so many people gravitate toward lifestyle influencers on social media in the first place. The relentlessly chic young moms and perpetually vacationing 20-somethings present an aspirational worldview. Then they recommend the products and services that help you achieve it. Once you find a couple of influencers whose tastes you like, they do the work of narrowing down all the available options to just those that adhere to your particular sensibility.

Professor Renata Salecl, author of *The Tyranny of Choice*, further explains this in a Guardian article, "Privatization of electricity did not bring the desired outcome – lesser prices, better service – however, it did contribute to the anxiety and feeling of guilt on the side of the consumers. We feel that it is our fault we are paying too much, and we are anxious that a better deal is just around the corner. However, while we are losing valuable time doing research on which provider to choose, we then stop short of actually making the choice." So we do nothing, and corporations gain more profits from our inaction. All of this shakes up the idea that human beings act in such a way that they maximize their well-being and minimize their pain. Salecl added, "People often act against their well-being. They also rarely make choices in a rational way."

How this impacts your decision making and ultimately taking

any sort of action to improve your life is quite devastating. It can result in decision fatigue, sticking to the default option, or even avoiding making a decision altogether. This especially happens when we are deciding in an area we are not knowledgeable enough about. This makes it so much more challenging for us to learn new things, take new actions that will improve our lives, and even prevent us from growing before we even had the chance to take just one step.

Schwartz summarizes why this happens and what this is precisely through the following two narrative aspects of choice:

1. **Analysis paralysis:** The more choices presented often leads to a worse user experience. The more options offered to us distract from the desired goal. Especially when there are calls to action, more is not better.

2. **Buyer's remorse:** Generally, the more choices you have, the worse you feel after you buy something. Why is that? Because your standards have been raised now that you have been presented with more options to choose from. Now, all you can think about is how much better your other options may have been for you.

In a New York Times article, *Too Many Choices: A Problem That Can Paralyze*, Benjamin Scheibehenne, a Professor at the Karlsruhe Institute of Technology (KIT), Institute for Information Systems and Marketing, explains the critical information we use to make our choices, "It might be too simple to conclude that too many choices are bad, just as it is wrong to assume that more choices are always better. It can depend on what information we're being given as we make those choices, the type of expertise we have to rely on, and how much importance we ascribe to each choice." So it's not just the overwhelming amount of choices. It's the confusion and polarization of choices. No one can deny the power and influence social media has.

It makes perfect sense based on what we've discussed and what you probably already know about how social media plays such a pivotal role in influencing lifestyle choices. But why is there so much conflict about the choices we make with purchases, social issues, and more? Why is there much more emotional pressure to make seemingly trivial choices? Social media directly impacts our decision making because it creates more connections to receive information and opinions. People tend to trust the opinions of participants in online networks in which they have chosen to participate.

If you see multiple people within your network traveling to luxury hotels or taking mirror selfies to showcase how good, they look (and even feel) that would influence you on many levels to eventually mimic the same thing. Influencers play a large role in this because they are people who, through their hard work and passion, have built a reputation for their expertise. These influencers have a sizable and trusted network of engaged fans and followers. Based on this trust, influencers create trends thus influencing perspectives on a variety of topics (like fashion choices, views on social issues, what a "good life should look like", etc.) and even influence the buying decisions of their followers. In *Change: The Power in the Periphery to Make Big Things Happen,* author Damon Centola offers even more insight in how this works. Centola used scientific studies to explore how beliefs, behaviors, and ideas spread through social networks for a popular audience.

What he discovered was something quite interesting. In one

experiment, he divided a group into two. The first group was *centralized,* where a small number of people, or perhaps just one person is at the *center* of the network. This person is connected to many other people in the *periphery.*

The second group was *egalitarian* – the opposite of a centralized network. In the egalitarian group, everyone has an equal number of contacts and therefore influence throughout the entire network. The key feature of this unbiased network is that new ideas and points of view can emerge from anywhere in the community and spread to everyone. The experiment revealed that within this network, views actually became much more moderate, and new ideas flourished. What was further discovered in these experiments with the centralized network group is that ideas were filtered through algorithms, or sometimes even blocked, by a robust social influencer.

You see, in social media, networks tend to always be centralized. The multitudes in the periphery of social networks have only a modest number of connections, while the few (influencers) are at the center of the network and are connected to nearly everyone. This puts these people into the powerful position of exerting a disproportionate level of *influence* over the group. This feature of social media is one of the main reasons why misinformation and fake news have become so pervasive.

In centralized networks, biased influencers have a disproportionate impact on their community—enabling small rumors and claims to become amplified into widespread misconceptions and false beliefs. Keep in mind influencers can be people, but they can also be companies as well. Both have much to gain in persuading you to think a certain way. In a centralized echo chamber, if the influencer in the middle shows even a small amount of partisan bias, it can become amplified throughout the entire group.

In egalitarian networks, ideas spread based on their quality. Not the person who's touting them. There is a lot of wisdom in network peripheries, in regular people with good ideas. When the social network enables those people to speak with each other, new thinking that challenges a group's biases can take hold and spread throughout the network.

What I like so much about the social experiment that Centola created is that he proved that we can still discover a way not to be so polarized. We may not necessarily be there yet because, after all, we do have nothing but centralized social media networks, and it seems to be a growing trend. That doesn't mean that we won't find a way to decentralize it or improve the situation. In the meantime, we can be more intentional about how we digest information by revisiting our learned principles from *The Maguire Method* to make sure we're not easily being influenced by others. With such an emphasis on building social influence, there is something to be said that, in reality, too many social media connections can increase your stress level.

For example, a report from the University of Edinburgh Business School stated that more Facebook friends causes more stress. Researchers also linked an abundance of social media connections to increased anxiety about offending people. This stress stemmed from people's desire to present a version of themselves that was acceptable to all their social media contacts. That stress can lead to word vomit on social posts about personal issues that could otherwise be kept private in hopes that someone can relate. Worse, a complete fabrication of someone's life in hopes of impressing you. We all do it in different ways or have someone close to us that does. The amount of stress that someone has can lead to depression, anxiety, and more.

I myself have experienced that type of stress as a social media influencer. At times, I've contemplated for hours about what I would write in a social media caption that would attract the most support. I have even gravitated towards specific restaurants so that I could snap a few photos of delicious dishes to share with my followers. I would do this without even giving a second thought about being present in the moment.

On a more serious note, I'm a very outspoken voice regarding social issues. This was spotlighted even more in 2020 when the recognition of the Black Lives Matter movement surged. I received some negative comments directed towards my social posts from targeted spam bots and naysayers (some were my followers, but, oddly enough, most were not), even though it was only a small amount of criticism. Probably around two out of ten comments. Those few criticisms made me reevaluate my own values and principles. That's how easily we can be destabilized and separated from our own values.

Negatively fueled social interactions were highlighted by a social media post I shared at the beginning of the Covid-19 pandemic. I simply wished everyone "Good Morning. Keep your head up." I do this all of the time. It's kind of my thing. This time, the first response I received was a swift "Fuck off." Even though the reactions to follow were more kind and supportive, it still caused me to overthink sharing social posts in general. Something so simple like this can become overwhelming. One way we can resolve this feeling of being overwhelmed is to apply minimalism to our lives.

This is an effective way to simplify our decision-making.

Applying minimalism will allow you the freedom to declutter your mind and reshape your environment. I learned this the hard way while going through a tough stretch with my ad agency. If you've never run your own business before, there are times when you feel euphoric and so fulfilled you're like an unstoppable juggernaut.

Other times you go through these rough patches where you feel like you're stuck in quicksand as an avalanche is barreling towards you. It can be terrifying if you don't know how to respond to times like these. During the best of times with my agency, tapping into the early stages of the Silicon Beach movement in Los Angeles rewarded us with quick success. From interviews in Forbes to keynote speeches at countless conventions, our presence was felt everywhere. At one point, I had thought I had it all.

Our ad agency was a primarily digital business. Nearly all of our leads and clients came from word of mouth and a fantastic online reputation. So, we never had to seek out new business. It would just come to us. So, you know when you get those email messages or offers that sound too good to be true? Well, we would receive those types of queries every day, and most of the time, they ended up being a long-term valued client.

With success like that, there was always something to do. Everything was urgent, from late-night texts, urgent emails, emergency phone calls, and meetings to last-minute changes on time-sensitive projects. There was this unrelenting feeling of never quite getting ahead but not falling behind if things went smoothly. But it's the perfect recipe for disaster when things don't go smoothly. Eventually, that's what happened.

During this time, Donald Trump became president, and with this came a new cloud of discomfort that hung over every professional encounter. There was always this constant air of anxiety, increasingly argumentative stances, and ultimately questions of if the values and principles were in alignment with our own. It was a domino effect. The unhappy clients were becoming more challenging to deal with. The happy ones were becoming more overbearing.

Even onboarding more prominent clients with enormous expectations became too much to handle. Our highest paying client had a troubling discovery of tax evasion that forced them to terminate our agreement early while skipping out on paying the penalty and monies owed. We were even scammed by a business lead. Then there was my private life with being a co-parent and struggling to keep my romantic relationship afloat. With every problem solved, there were two more at my doorstep.

Ultimately, all of the pressures and life challenges I faced were too much to handle. My heartbreaking breakup, followed by the eventual closing of our agency, was gut-wrenching. Money troubles soon followed, and things kept getting worse with no end in sight. It got to a point where I had to choose between getting gas or groceries for my daughter and myself. I had to borrow money from my ex-wife, family, friends, and even predatory loans. This would be just the beginning of a long season of learning lessons.

Having nothing, having to "start over", was a truly humbling experience. I tried to climb out of my hole by scaling back, managing my smaller client base, renting out my home on Airbnb, and doing anything I could to survive. One day, one of my best friends came to check on me and took me out to a concert.

When he dropped me off, I noticed my car was missing. It had been repossessed. Eventually, I would get my car back, but I had to make the tough decision to move out of my home. I put most of my belongings in a storage unit and moved into a small room in the house. My daughter and I shared a bed, a bathroom, and a closet. There was a lot of soul-searching during this time.

I was stripped away from most of my choices and not a day went by where there weren't tears flowing and me asking how did I go from having it all to nothing at all? I asked all the wrong questions that only fueled my insecurities. I got all the wrong answers when I did this. So, even when I took action, it was unfocused and lacked clarity. That's how I discovered to nail down the steps of the first two principles of *The Maguire Method* that I shared with you.

I learned that when you're cornered with nothing to lose, even at that moment, you have a choice. You can choose to surrender or fight back. I chose the latter with more clarity and intention. I took massive action, and yes! I eventually climbed out of the hole I was in. I was even able to get to a place in my life that was even better than where I was during my best years.

Except for this time, everything was different. I was different. Then came the moment to finally get my belongings out of storage. When I was finally there, I just stood there quietly—staring ahead at the expensive furniture I once owned, clothes, hoverboards, TVs, etc. All of it felt meaningless—all of it.

After all, I experienced what life was like when I didn't have it. I grabbed a few heirlooms and critical things I needed. Then I gave everything else to the movers right then and there. Anything left over. I had the Salvation Army come and pick it up.

I remember thinking how fearful I once was of things that didn't matter when I struggled to stay afloat. Hell, where were the Joneses when I needed them? Who cares? I became more interested in new ideas. I'm not necessarily telling you that you need to go out and get rid of everything. I am telling you to rethink what and who matters the most to you.

I leaned more into a life of minimalism and investing in experiences with the people that mean the most to me. It wasn't massive action alone that helped me. It was discovering ways how I could create and apply our first two principles to my way of life. I didn't just learn to dream again. I learned how to make those dreams a reality. Even though the darkest of times, we can persevere in ascending to heights we never thought possible.

We live in a world where we are consciously and subconsciously fighting off depression, anxiety, and stress from the moment we wake up to the moment we go to sleep. It's no wonder why it's challenging to find peace in an otherwise chaotic world. Even shutting things out or off is only a temporary solution, which is why we must reshape things even more and not avoid the storm. Instead, gear up for it and then go through it.

Burnout has become an increasing and often-discussed part of our lives over the last decade. Even with all of the action we can take to overcome the odds, there is a growing trend of burnout that seems to be unavoidable. The term "burnout" was first used in the 70's by two psychologists, Herbert Freudenberger and Christina Maslach, who independently studied this phenomenon in social service and health workers. They specifically targeted these sectors due to the high volume of human interaction and the chronic stress experienced daily. They discovered that burnout is a psychological syndrome of emotional exhaustion, depersonalization, and reduced personal accomplishments that can occur among individuals who feel overworked in some capacity.

Typically, the key aspects of this response are:

- Overwhelming exhaustion
- Feelings of cynicism and detachment
- A sense of ineffectiveness
- Lack of accomplishment

The most common sources of burnout among adults step from work, money, and health. In the United States alone, levels of stress vary from person to person depending on a variety of factors that can influence your feelings, including employment status, age, income, and ethnicity. So, if you feel like your best isn't good enough and you're exhausted even trying, you are not alone.

Burnout can slow us down while we're trying to transform our lives for the better and even, in some cases, lead to death. It's hard to find the energy to do anything when you have already spent it, right? The hard truth is that burnout is unavoidable. But if we understand how it works more, we can discover new ways to lessen its impact on our lives. To even better understand what burnout looks like, look at its four stages below:

1. **Dissatisfaction:** The first burnout stage is characterized by a lack of awareness that anything's wrong. You may have some minor thoughts of discomfort or a subtle gut feeling that something's "off." You most likely write it off as just being a part of life, though.

2. **Subconscious Disregard:** This stage of burnout introduces increasingly uncomfortable thoughts and emotions. You're noticeably irritable and anxious. Repetitive mental patterns start nagging you, signaling that something's off-balance. At this point, your subconscious begins actively working out ways to manage the stress. Dysfunction

at work may lead to getting annoyed with your partner. You may start experiencing feelings of jealousy of your friends' success, silently project self-righteous judgments, or even blame everyone around for how you feel.

3. **Anxious Exhaustion:** This is when burnout symptoms manifest in your behavior. Feeling overwhelmed, exhausted, and worried feels too big to swallow. So, you start relying on one or more numbing techniques to defer discomfort. This is when procrastination enters the picture. You attempt to conserve your energy.

    You're late a lot. You'll do anything but the very thing you need to do, and you certainly do not derive joy from what you need to do. You experience two cycles: numbing (or overstimulating) yourself to power through challenges and then feeling extremely low as a result. There's no balance or peace during this cycle. Even when you're supposed to be resting, you can't help but think about all the things you need to do. Can you relate?

4. **Habitual Burnout:** Living in a chronic state of excessive stress can lead to dangerous places. The most common symptom of this final burnout stage is a complete physical shut-down or uncontrollable anxiety, also known as panic attacks. This is a pretty frightening stage of burnout because it can lead to a feeling of failure, helplessness, and crisis. This can ultimately lead to suicidal thoughts, exhaustion, and depression. We don't want to get to this point as it gets increasingly hard to get out of.

We should aim to get no further past the second stage of burnout. If blow past that stage, try some fresh techniques in our reflections principle to be mindful of the following burnout triggers so you have a better understanding of how to combat them effectively. I have listed five ways that you can use if you're experiencing burnout or getting close to:

1. **Workload:** You can be more productive when you are working on a workload that aligns with your capacity. A manageable workload allows you more opportunities to rest and recover. It's also an avenue for you to develop yourself and grow. That's not the case when you are overloaded with work or are facing unrealistic deadlines set by your boss. You will lose the chance of regaining your balance.

2. **Absence of autonomy:** If you feel that you don't have access to vital resources and even a say in various decisions that affect your professional and personal life, it can impact your health. For instance, do you receive calls from your boss all night? Do you have what it takes to influence your work or home environment? Does your family saddle you with responsibilities beyond your capacity?

3. **Environment:** In some instances, some of you can't choose your work environment or even the people around you. But you can always optimize your environment. Your environment can upgrade your engagement or downgrade it, so always ask yourself, who do you collaborate with? How trusting and supportive are your work relationships?

4. **Reward:** If the intrinsic and extrinsic rewards don't align with your level of effort, you may begin to feel a lack of motivation to exert any effort at all. For instance, you may need a face-time with your employer, positive feedback, or

an increase in your compensation. Find out which reward makes you feel appreciated and seek avenues to receive more of it.

5. **Values Mismatch:** If you are working in an organization or have clients that don't share your same values, you will continue to see a decline in your level of motivation. For instance, if you strongly believe in making an impact first, before money, you will experience burnout on the job in an organization that prioritizes money over impact.

Since the global pandemic, quite a number of people have often experienced the third stage of burnout. We never want to get to stage four. Burnout can happen to anyone, even those who enjoy their jobs and careers. The impact of burnout can be deadly. It increases your moodiness, strains your relationships, thins out your prefrontal cortex (the part of the brain responsible for cognitive functioning), weakens your memory and attention spans, and even shares similar damage to someone who has experienced intense traumas.

Remember, burnout doesn't just show up overnight. It builds itself gradually with every task. With every small favor, you half-heartedly accept despite your current workload, health, and values, you're working toward burnout. We know the symptoms, the causes, and their effects. How can we recover, recharge, and ultimately rebalance ourselves?

First, try the tactics you learned in our first two principles of *The Maguire Method*. Use our first principle to ask great questions to yourself if you're feeling burnt out. Here are a few questions to get you started:

- Am I enjoying the work I do?
- Am I receiving enough support for what I'm doing?
- Am I currently experiencing a good work-life balance?
- Are there opportunities for growth from what I'm doing?

Next, apply our reflections principle to utilize some of the strategies and exercises laid out for you to re-calibrate yourself. Then, try the following tips to tackle burnout:

Fuck 'em. Say "No": When you recover from severe burnout, don't take on any additional work or projects. Don't repeat the mistakes you made before. It's okay to set boundaries. It's okay to simply say one magical word… "No".

Take regular breaks: Our brains are not wired to sustain extended periods of attention, which is why focusing for too long on a task can lower our motivation and the performance needed to complete our tasks. The solution to this is to have short breaks throughout our day. This is the perfect time for leg stretches, calls with loved ones, walks in the park, etc. Basically, anything that moves you away from your computer and allows you the space to regroup your mind. Don't shy away from taking vacations either.

Team up with an accountability partner: Always opt to have an accountability partner (or multiple) who will help motivate you to succeed with whatever it is that you're working on. Doing this will not just help you decrease burnout when you're already feeling it but it can also help it not be so severe in the first place. Whether you are trying to excel at a project that will earn you a promotion at work or you're making an attempt at a pressure-free hobby like learning how to cook a particular type of food, an accountability partner will help you along your journey.

Burnout recovery is best when you don't have to use it. Taking action is what will transform your life. All you have to keep in mind is that with just one step, there is progress. The best decision that you could ever make in your life is to put your words into action and manifest the life you always wanted for yourself. You never know how one thing you can do can impact someone else.

When you put in the work or the action for yourself, and you're doing it with positivity and good health, it's almost like you're sending out a signal to others. It's infectious, and people are always receptive to that signal. That's why the first two steps of *The Maguire Method* are so necessary.

When you're intentional about how you want to see the world and how you want to make an impact in this world, then it seamlessly slips into how you're going to act. For some of us, it may seem foreign. For others, it may seem all right, but in any situation, it simply takes time for you to see the full effect of things. Always remember that all it takes is one step. That one step leads to empowerment and freedom in ways that you didn't think were possible.

CHAPTER ELEVEN

Your Perfect Day

Establishing the tone of your day the right way sets you up for success and joy. When you start off with a good rhythm, it doesn't matter what life throws at you. It gives you more opportunities to deal with it from a better perspective. It's just as easy to set the tone in a shitty way. One isn't more complex than the other. Why not try it the way that's more inclined to set you up for success? Everything from your environment to the people in your daily life also plays a vital role in your productivity, happiness, and success.

In our first two principles, we discovered ways in which we can sharpen our minds and spirits. With that in mind, we are now able to shift our mindset to more of one of abundance. You can clearly understand our intentions with the actions we take. You will learn that from taking massive action to even the smallest action you may take for granted will produce amazing results for you.

This abundant mindset also helps us establish the right tone to dive into how we begin each day. Spiritual leader Thich Nhat Hanh once said, "Because of your smile, you make life more beautiful." So why not start every day with a smile?

Is it because… you have nothing to smile about? Are you anxious about work you have to rush off to? Do you feel like runover shit from having one too many drinks the night before? Not a morning person? All of the above can be true, and you can still start your day with a smile.

Psychologists discovered that people smile because they feel happy. It's also true that people feel so glad when they smile. This means that you don't have to experience anything positive to be joyful. To be clear, I'm not a morning person. Anybody that's ever woken up next to me can vouch for that.

For years, I was grumpy as hell in the mornings. The first time I ever experimented with waking up with a smile on my face, I felt like an asshole. On the second day, I asked myself, "What's the point of this?" (which is an example of a bad question.) On the third day, I was already over it. I forced myself to do it anyway.

On the fourth day, I laughed out loud about how absurd it was that I was forcing myself to smile every morning. Each day I did it afterward. It was my own inside joke to myself. I just thought it was ludicrous. I was forcing myself to start my day with a smile. Well, before long, others noticed I was always smiling in the mornings. I saw how people interacted with me was much more pleasant and open.

Finally, one day I went into a cafe to order a coffee, and the barista commented, "Look at you smiling. I wish I could be a morning person." Smiling is just the beginning. A simple smile goes a long way but setting the tone of your day with a morning ritual that works best for you is a life changer. You always do what works best for you, but if you establish a morning ritual, you have just unlocked a secret next level.

The world is chaotic and unpredictable, and we have to create ways to organize the chaos to find peace in our own world. A great morning ritual does that for you because it sets the tone of your day by your own standards. Whatever life throws at you (no doubt it will), you can handle it better. Of course, you can always shake up your morning routine if it becomes too stale. I think there are at least two things you should do every morning as a part of your ritual to help you stay grounded and establish the tone of your day.

My "secret sauce" is to get a head start on your day before everyone else in your home. The first step is the one you're most likely dreading… wake up early. At least 30 minutes before you already do now. This gives you the space to calmly begin your day with clarity and liberates you from the chaos that will come with the day as it unfolds.

I'm the first one awake in my home, and it gives me the time I need to clear my thoughts. I like to journal over a cup of coffee and visualize my day. I often read the trades and listen to podcasts. I keep it really mellow. This works for me. You always do what works best for you.

Out of nowhere, my daughter bursts into the kitchen excitedly. One morning, I went about my morning routine. It was a rainy morning, and I was sipping some fresh hot coffee and reading a book. I even had jazz playing in the background. I don't even listen to jazz. I was just setting the mood.

She was going on a field trip and had rapid-fire questions for me if I took care of this or that. Her teacher said this and that. Before I could get a word in, she bumped me, and I spilled coffee all over my shirt. It burned like hell, and I jumped to my feet, knocking over my mug. The mug smashed into pieces, and my coffee spilled all over the floor. My daughter rushed to help, but she ran through the spilled coffee.

Chaos erupted in the Johnson home within seconds. I went to double-check that my cell phone was dry, and when I did, I saw at that exact moment an incoming text from my most important client, "PLEASE CONTACT ME WHEN YOU CAN. WE HAVE A VERY BIG…" At that moment, I burst out into… laughter.

Because I had just a little bit of an extra head start and was intentional about waking up early and setting the town of my day, it allowed me to be proactive on my own terms. So, I could respond calmly and thoughtfully if anything else were to happen after that. Also, I had the time to clean up, get my daughter ready for school, and promptly respond to the incoming text. There was no rushing or reason to get upset.

I had the extra time I needed to get things sorted out. Whenever chaos unfolds all at once in a "when it rains, it pours" way, it just usually means you need to slow down. Other times it means you should be more present. More often than not, we give too much power to things that happen out of our control. We should never just easily give our power away like that. Remember, life has just as many challenges as rewards.

For the record, the rest of that day was pretty awful. It was simply just one day, though. There were still victories through-out the day, and I still remember that magical start I had before chaos unfolded. Getting into a nice rhythm of an inspiring morning routine is one thing but tackling an entire day is an-other. Once our day gets underway, it will be filled with chal-lenges, distractions, ups, and downs. Even on a "perfect day", you'll have low periods.

If you find it challenging to find the right time or energy to take action, remember that this is a process. If we're intentional about that process, we'll create more chances for getting what you need and want in life. Just doing one of the following actions is going to get you one step closer to achieving the level of success, productivity, and happiness that you desire. If you're able to tackle everything listed, that's awesome. However, this isn't created for you to be an overachiever.

I'm aiming to help you have a more rewarding life, and you can do that by doing what works for you and you alone. As you read the following, I want you to think about how you can take just one of the following actions to craft a masterful day of actions that will deliver impact.

Reshape Your Environment: Your environment influences your mood and behavior, so shape your environment to bring out the best in yourself. Many times, we may struggle with motivation, energy, or even feel downright depressed, not knowing that there is something out of sorts in our environment.

Environmental cues are objects in or aspects of our surroundings that trigger specific thoughts and desires, causing us to think or behave in certain ways. It's little things that we often take for granted and go unnoticed. For example, if your phone is always within arm's reach in eyesight, of course, you can't help but want to check it more often than you should. If your desk is messy and you often feel disorganized, now is the time to connect the dots on how one can affect the other.

It doesn't matter if you set out to complete a task with the best intentions. If your environment dictates otherwise, you're doomed. We look around ourselves at other people, objects, and the way our environment is set up to determine how we should act. Reshaping your environment can apply to everything. Even changing the little details of your environment makes a big difference when we're forming habits and reinforcing the actions in our lives.

By reshaping your environment and creating a configuration that empowers and motivates you, you'll see how big of a change that makes. For example, I read that having plants in your home or office can boost your mood. So, I filled my home with plants. I loved the vibrant energy they brought to my house. I even gained fulfillment from watering the plants and nurturing them.

Having the plants allowed me to keep to a consistent routine, and I could literally see the progress I made as the plants continued to blossom and grow. After a while, that became boring for me, so I again reshaped my environment by rearranging the plants in different areas of my home to change up the decor. That's the thing. Your environment should be on your terms. You can reshape your environment whenever you want.

Fill your space with inspirational imagery, and decorate your home with inspiring sticky notes for the rest of your inhabitants. Fill your office area with bright colors and request to DJ the office playlist for a period of time during the day. Declutter your space and shape it into a space that makes you feel motivated. Put time limits on your web browsing use.

Change your cell phone wallpaper. Do as much as you want or as little as you want. Change it up routinely or leave it the way it is as long as it makes you feel energized and inspired. Whatever works for you works for you. Little things like this make a big difference.

Annihilate your most important task first: Destroy your day's most important task before anything else. This task should be from your goal-related to-do list that will have the most impact on achieving your goal. This task makes other things on your to-do list obsolete, faster, or more accessible. Instead of aiming for ten steps to a process that you think you need to achieve a goal, choose the one step that obliterates the other ones. If you're not sure how to determine what action you should take, simply rate your tasks according to the impact they have on achieving your main goal.

Always choose the one with the highest (potential) impact, whether it's a personal goal (lose weight, run that marathon, find a new apartment) or a professional goal (start a blog, get that promotion, change careers). It's usually not whatever lurks in your inbox or that "urgent" work task you need to do. You can do that right after this one thing. If your job is mostly about dealing with urgent tasks, structure your day in a way that lets you achieve your most important tasks for yourself first. When you're able to plan ahead as a part of your morning routine you can do it with more ease.

Use your moods to your advantage: Our moods shift and change throughout the day, and if we can understand when that happens, we can use that to your advantage. According to Daniel Pink's book, *When: The Scientific Secrets of Perfect Timing*, regardless of your chronotype (your "type", whether you're a morning or evening person, is known as your *chronotype*), when your mood is low, it's usually the best time for you to do more administrative work (ex: answering emails, filling out expense reports, etc.) or routine stuff (dumping the trash, washing the dishes, etc.). During recovery, which is later in the day for most people, our mood boosts back up, but you're less vigilant. Pink explains, "This combination of enhanced mood while being less analytical makes a good time for brainstorming and creative work." All human beings have a natural circadian rhythm, the 24-hour cycle that governs our physiology. This cycle causes you to feel a certain level of wakefulness or tiredness around the same time each day.

Why We Sleep by Matthew Walker is clear to point out that not all of us are on the same circadian rhythm. For some people, their peak of wakefulness arrives early in the day, and their peak of sleepiness comes early at night. There are "morning types" that account for about 40% of the population. These people tend to wake up around dawn and are happy to do so. In fact, they function optimally at this time of day.

Other people are "evening types" and account for about 30% of the population. These people prefer going to bed late and waking up late the following morning. The remaining 30% of the population falls somewhere between a morning and evening type. Your type is primarily determined by genetics. If you're a night owl, it's likely that one or both of your parents is a night owl.

You can best discover what your chronotype is and find out how you want to best organize your day by trying one or both of the following tactics:

First, answer the following three questions:

1. What time do you usually go to bed?
2. What time do you usually wake up?
3. What is the midpoint between those two times?

For example, if you normally go to bed at 2 a.m. and wake up at 10 a.m., your midpoint is 6 a.m. The second tactic to try is to keep track of your daily routine. First, set your alarm to go off every 90 minutes while you're awake, then note what you're doing, how mentally alert do you feel, and how energetic you feel. Do this for a full week.

At the end of the week, you should see trends when you're feeling the most and least alert. Use that to determine how your internal clock ebbs and flows over the course of the day. Then simply plan accordingly.

4 Hours of Peak Performance: According to Productivity researcher Anders Ericsson, top performers in various fields seem to max out at four hours per day of deep work. On average, you have 3-4 hours of deep flow state work every day. "Flow state" is when you have a long stretch of unbroken concentration and focus. This is valuable, meaningful, and rare but can be developed especially if you practice the steps in the core *Maguire Method* principles.

Cal Newport, the author of *Deep Work*, writes, "Three to four hours a day, five days a week, of uninterrupted and carefully directed concentration, it turns out, can produce a lot of valuable output." Finding 3-4 hours of deep work is easier said than done. Once it becomes a habit, it's hard to break. I also think for all of us, "deep work" might be defined as something different. For me, "deep work" might be that I have back-to-back meetings that I need to be 100% locked in for.

Maybe for you, it's programming, or for someone else, it's research or perfecting a dance routine. In any scenario, it's hyper-focused work. A study by the IZA Institute of Labor Economics analyzed half a million exams taken by university students in the United Kingdom at three different times of day: 9:00 a.m., 1:30 p.m., and 4:30 p.m. Based on five years of exam scores and an average of six exams per student, the researchers found that "peak performance" usually happens during the 1:30 p.m. slot. There's some wiggle room, obviously.

Maybe you're too "hangry" at lunchtime to even think about work or tend to get your best work done right after that first cup of coffee hits at 9 a.m. Find your sweet spot. When you do, get in your deep work state.

Body In Motion: It doesn't matter how you do it or even when you do it. Motion is everything. It's actually a secret ingredient to happiness and success we usually overlook. Move a muscle, change a thought. Changing behavior is the key to feeling better. Here are a five standout benefits that really spotlight why moving your body is so important and enhance your mental fortitude along with small steps you can take:

1. **Muscles:** You have more than 600 muscles in your body that contribute to about 40% of your total body weight. You are strengthening your muscles by moving, which improves stability, balance, and coordination. Stretching also helps maintain your muscle health.

2. **Bones:** Movement helps build more durable, denser bones. With bone-building activities like resistance training (weights), weight-bearing exercises (jogging, walking, hiking), and balance training (yoga), you can better support your bone density.

3. **Joints:** Moving your joints encourages flexibility and range of motion. Yoga is a great exercise to work out your joints because it is all about body awareness. You increase coordination and balance by being aware of how you

move. So you're compelled to pay attention to each movement while doing yoga exercises.

4. **Brain:** Walking 30-40 minutes a day three times per week can help regrow the brain structures linked to cognitive decline in older adults. If you are working from home or tend to sit more often, be sure to make an effort to take walks.

5. **Heart:** According to the British Heart Foundation, we can avoid around 10,000 fatal heart attacks each year if we keep fit. Cycling is a great exercise to improve your heart health. In fact, regular cycling can cut your risk of heart disease by 50%.

Spend quality time with loved ones: Make time for the people you care about. Never be too busy to check in on someone or make time for your loved ones. By doing so, not only are you increasing your sense of belonging and purpose, but you're also boosting your happiness and reducing your stress. When you nurture your community, it helps prevent loneliness and gives you a chance to offer needed companionship, too.

In one of the longest studies of adult life, a Harvard Study of Adult Development studied the lives of 724 men for 78 years. Although this study centered on white men as it has gone over the years, the study has included people of color and women, including the participants' spouses, partners, and family members of the test subjects. Investigators survey the group every two years about their physical and mental health, professional lives, friendships, and marriages. The subjects also do periodic in-person interviews, medical exams, blood tests, and brain scans.

Psychiatrist Robert J. Waldinger, the study's Director and

Principal Investigator shared some of the major lessons in a popular TED Talk, *What makes a good life? Lessons from the longest study on happiness.* Waldinger said, "It's the quality of your relationships that matters." Researchers found that when their subjects looked back on their lives, people most often reported their time spent with others as the most meaningful. It was also the part of their lives of which they were the proudest.

Spending time with other people made study subjects happier on a day-to-day basis, and in particular, time with a partner or spouse seemed to buffer them against the mood dips that come with aging's physical pains and illnesses. "Loneliness kills", Waldinger says. "It's as powerful as smoking or alcoholism". Waldinger especially noted, "The surprising finding is that our relationships and how happy we are in our relationships have a powerful influence on our health. Taking care of your body is important, but tending to your relationships is a form of self-care too."

It didn't matter about anyone's social class, wealth, fame (some were even former U.S. presidents), IQ, or even genes. When George Vaillant, a psychiatrist, and professor at Harvard Medical School, spoke about the study, he further stated, "The only thing that really matters in life are your relationships to other people."

I often refer to my "Impact List" (a shortlist of family, friends, and colleagues that have a huge impact on my life). I'll tell you more in detail on how you can make this list in our last principle. This list is incredibly helpful because I use it to keep track of how often I check in with loved ones. It helps me stay accountable and tapped in especially when I'm dealing with my busy schedule. I always want to prioritize my personal relationships and this is one way to make sure I'm doing that.

So, reconcile with an old friend. Send a text check-in to some-one you care about. Have dinner with your family. Go for a walk with your best friend. Send a meme to your favorite co-worker. If you're the type that is the one always reaching out to someone, that's okay too. Just put in the effort to surround yourself with the ones you love. To sum it up, you'll live a happier and longer life when you make time for your people.

Eat to live, not live to eat: Choosing a healthy diet that works best for you will always pay off in the long run. You'll have more energy, manage stress better, and even feel better about yourself. Not to mention, you'll look great. First, you must be proactive about creating a diet plan that works best for you. Prioritize this so you can be intentional about what you put into your body. Then make your own meal plans.

Avoid "cheat days" altogether and instead, embrace a lifestyle that allows you to be more strategic with when and how much you eat. If you choose to graze all day long and don't have time to seek healthy options every time, it's going to make eating much more difficult. Instead, choose larger meals less frequently.

When you eat out, choose healthier options that fit into your diet plan. To avoid overeating, consider even splitting a meal with a friend. You can even ask for a smaller portion or put half of the plate in a to-go box for another time. Even gas stations and convenience shops often carry simple snacks like nuts, jerky, and fresh fruit that you can get in a pinch. If you're grabbing a bite at a fast-food restaurant, remember there are usually offerings of fresh salads, soups, and bun less burger options.

You will have to make an extra effort to find a good meal or even prepare a little in advance, but it can be done. I used to cook my meals on Sunday evenings. I even made it a fun ritual. I would put on music and prepare 3-4 various types of meals that I could pack away and eat throughout the week. Instead of turning it into a chore or something else I had to do, I had fun with it. This ended up saving me time and gave me more space to be intentional about what I put into my body.

Other days of the week, I would eat out with family or friends. When I did, I always tried to order meals we could share. I would learn that it wasn't just a healthy move for my body but also a fun bonding activity with people I care about while even discovering new foods at times.

Use "I am" positive affirmations: Practicing affirmations activates the reward system in your brain. When you know you have the ability to manage stress and other life difficulties, it boosts your confidence and self-empowerment. State your affirmations in the present tense with "I am." "I am" statements make your affirmations more powerful, resulting in a stronger faith in your own abilities. For example, "I am smart as all hell, and I will nail that presentation tomorrow."

If you add your goals to your affirmations, it can do wonders. The secret to using positive affirmations is to use a memorable phrase, quote, or statement that is credible and achievable for yourself. Affirmations are designed to promote behavior leading to a positive result for yourself.

Learn something new: We finally live in a time where most of the things we have questions about we can find some sort of answers to. It doesn't matter if it's stupid, mundane, significant, or exis-tential. You should always carve out a little time for yourself every day to learn something new. This can be from a book, the internet, your family member, a friend, or even observing a life experience that impacted you. Be hungry and eager to keep learning.

Research shows learning something new improves your brain health. When you learn something new, you are exercising your brain, which can help build new cells and connections between cells. This improves cognitive functions such as concentration, attention to detail, memory recall, and problem-solving. It also reduces the chance of developing dementia. Take the time to pursue knowledge, especially on topics you previously had no interest in.

When you do this, you might just discover something you might not have previously known. For example, my time at Mattel sharpened my skills as a storyteller and marketer. I can tell you from memory recall, random dates of when the first Barbie commercial aired to how toy marketing has evolved since then. This actually sharpened my skills as a storyteller and marketer. It's also fun to bring up random facts at cocktail parties. Be intentional about learning and reap the benefits.

True life examples of successful families, relationships, careers, wealth, and anyone who made their dreams come true are inspiring. Learning a true-life success story would also be handy as something new you should learn. You can do this by exploring biographies, documentaries, essays, and more. Something to keep in mind is that success stories are not meant to be copied, mimicked, or plagiarized. They are intended to provide you with some tips, strategies, insight, and answers to some of the things that you're trying to do for yourself.

If you're unsure how you're going to be a successful CEO, why don't you just see how other successful CEOs became successful? What did they all have in common? If you want to be the world's most fabulous chef, why not read the biographies of the world's greatest chefs?

Take a digital screen timeout: On average, people check their phones 150 times daily. Although this compulsive behavior is seen as a way to cope with stress and keep yourself up-to-date, we already know the impact it can have on your life. When you wake up, resist the urge to hop on your phone. Resist the urge to turn on your TV. Avoid your computer. Use your morning routine and reshape your environment to avoid digital screens altogether.

Responding to your digital screens activates a part of your brain that makes you reactive. It's one of the sneaky reasons why sometimes you feel so overwhelmed or your brain is mush throughout the day. Even checking your phone or inbox thirty minutes into your morning after your morning ritual is better than checking it the first thing in the morning when you wake up. One tactic I use all the time that I would highly recommend for you is to set up alarm notifications, time limits, and friendly reminders for yourself of when you can and cannot use your digital screens. This will help you get into the habit of not being so tempted.

Take a nap: Scientific studies have shown that a short rest can help you feel more alert, increase creativity, boost productivity, reduce stress, boost your immune system, improve your memory, increase your learning ability, give you more clarity, and make you happier. A short nap of 10-20 minutes is precisely enough shut-eye to reap the many restorative benefits of napping. Don't fall for the "sleep when I'm dead" banner. Instead, be sure to get plenty of rest, and you'll live a longer, healthier life.

Give yourself sweet reminders: Do one thing that reminds you how small you are in the universe. This will help keep you grounded and keep things in perspective. Observe the world around you. Do this with the intention. Do it alone. Watch the people around you. Notice your surroundings. Remind yourself you are a part of a grander design.

Reward Yourself: It's important to reward yourself every single day. When you're rewarding yourself, do something that refreshes your energy and soothes you. No matter what that might be, big or small. Make sure it's something relaxing where you can truly unwind. Always feel free to mix it up on a daily basis. Find ways to reward yourself where you don't need any sort of external validation or anyone else's company.

This is just for you. Here are a few suggestions that have been known to help you get started: listening to music, streaming television, watching a film, curating music playlists, reading books, listening to podcasts, playing a game, a fun physical activity, decluttering your life, sex, masturbation, organizing your desk, clean your space, journal, go to your favorite hangout spot, get quality some time with nature, or just simply take a walk. There is only one requirement. Whatever it is that you're doing, it must bring a smile to your face and joy.

I also mentioned streaming something or watching a movie as a fun reward for yourself, but like all things, do it in moderation. Try to ease up on the gas with binge-watching anything. A 2017 study by the University of Toledo's Department of Health and Recreation found that binge-watching TV or movies can increase anxiety symptoms and disrupt sleep. The study also found that participants who watched more than two hours of television each night displayed higher levels of depression than those who had shorter viewing times. The study also suggests that binge-watching can involve obsessive behavior.

This can involve symptoms such as lack of control, damaging health and social effects, feelings of guilt, and neglect of duties. It has to do with the rapid changes in images, sounds, and actions that your brain processes while you're passively receiving information. You aren't interacting with what you're seeing in the way you would when playing a video game or researching something online. So, if you like watching TV or movies, it might be good to cap it at two hours.

Pay it forward: Pass on your lessons learned. Share them on social media, email, in person, or whatever works best for you. Just pass it on. If just one person shares knowledge gained, imagine how powerful of an impact that will make in the world. Be intentional about how you can give back to others. It's a straightforward way of contributing to your community. If you can contribute in other ways, like through donations (time or money) and providing level-up opportunities for someone who needs (and deserves it), do that too.

Respect your night routine: Have as much respect for your night routine as your morning routine. There is something about a night routine that is uniquely special. How you end, your day is just as important as how you begin it. Even if you have a bad day, you can finish it in a good way. If you live alone, it's easier to have a consistent evening routine for yourself, but it's still manageable even if you don't.

Include one or any of the mentioned actions as a part of your evening routine, like spending quality time with loved ones, rewarding yourself, etc. The key ingredient isn't the sleep part. It's actually how you close out your day before you drift off to nighty nighttime.

Get some rest: When that time finally comes, the National Sleep Foundation advises that healthy adults need between 7 and 9 hours of sleep per night. Babies, young children, and teenagers need even more rest to enable their growth and development. People over 65 should also get 7 to 8 hours per night. We know by now the fantastic health benefits of sleep, but we should also recognize what happens if we don't get enough rest.

A 2018 study of more than 10,000 people shows that the body's ability to function declines if sleep isn't in the seven to eight hour range. If you're having trouble getting rest, this is also where you can apply our laid-out steps and strategies in our first two core principles. Your goal is to declutter your mind and be calm before you get to bed. Let's say you're like me and have trouble getting to sleep. Instead of drifting off to sleep, you're scrolling through your social media feed. That's pretty common.

But, like I stated before, it would be a smart move for you to just keep your mobile device out of sight. Falling asleep in front of your TV is also pretty common. Currently, there's not a lot of research on using it as a sleep aid. According to a National Sleep Foundation poll, 60% of Americans watch TV right before falling asleep. A survey by LG Electronics reported that 61% of people fall asleep with the television on.

So, for some of you, it is a part of your nightly ritual. Perhaps some of you find the background noise relaxing or think it actually helps you fall asleep. The scientific intel that is available so far seems to be a mixed bag. One study published in the Journal of Behavioral Sleep Medicine found that using media of any kind as a sleep aid puts a damper on sleep quality. Another study linked internet use to the worst sleep quality but not necessarily television use.

When you set the volume low enough on your TV, the effect might be similar to using a white noise machine. It's when the volume level of our TV is loud enough to drown out the thoughts bombarding your racing mind but not so loud that it prevents your body from going into sleep mode. That ambient noise could actually decrease the amount of time it takes you to fall asleep. Even putting on a TV episode or movie that you've already seen multiple times can offer a sense of familiarity and comfort.

This is especially the case if what you're watching is lighter in nature, like those old episodes of *Friends*, *The Office*, *Martin*, etc. This will make it less likely than a new binge-worthy show to trigger an emotional response that will keep you awake. You will help lessen their harmful effects by tweaking your pre-sleep TV habits. You could even go so far as to set your television to turn off automatically at a specific time to cut out the light after you sleep. Make sure you don't become too dependent on TV as a sleep aid, either.

The best-recommended strategy overall is to simply whittle down your TV use and institute new calming bedtime behaviors like reading, meditating, or journaling. Having a variety of sleep-promoting options up your sleeve can help you steer clear of becoming too reliant on any one habit. This might increase your chances of scoring a quality night's sleep no matter the environment you're snoozing in. If you can find time to apply any of these tactics to your everyday schedule, you'll discover the many benefits to your life. You'll find that you will have more time to invest in the things that you actually care about.

Remember you want to take the action that matters to you based on your values, principles, and boundaries. When you apply all of our core principles to your life and make it a part of your habitual routine, you will find happiness and success.

HABITS

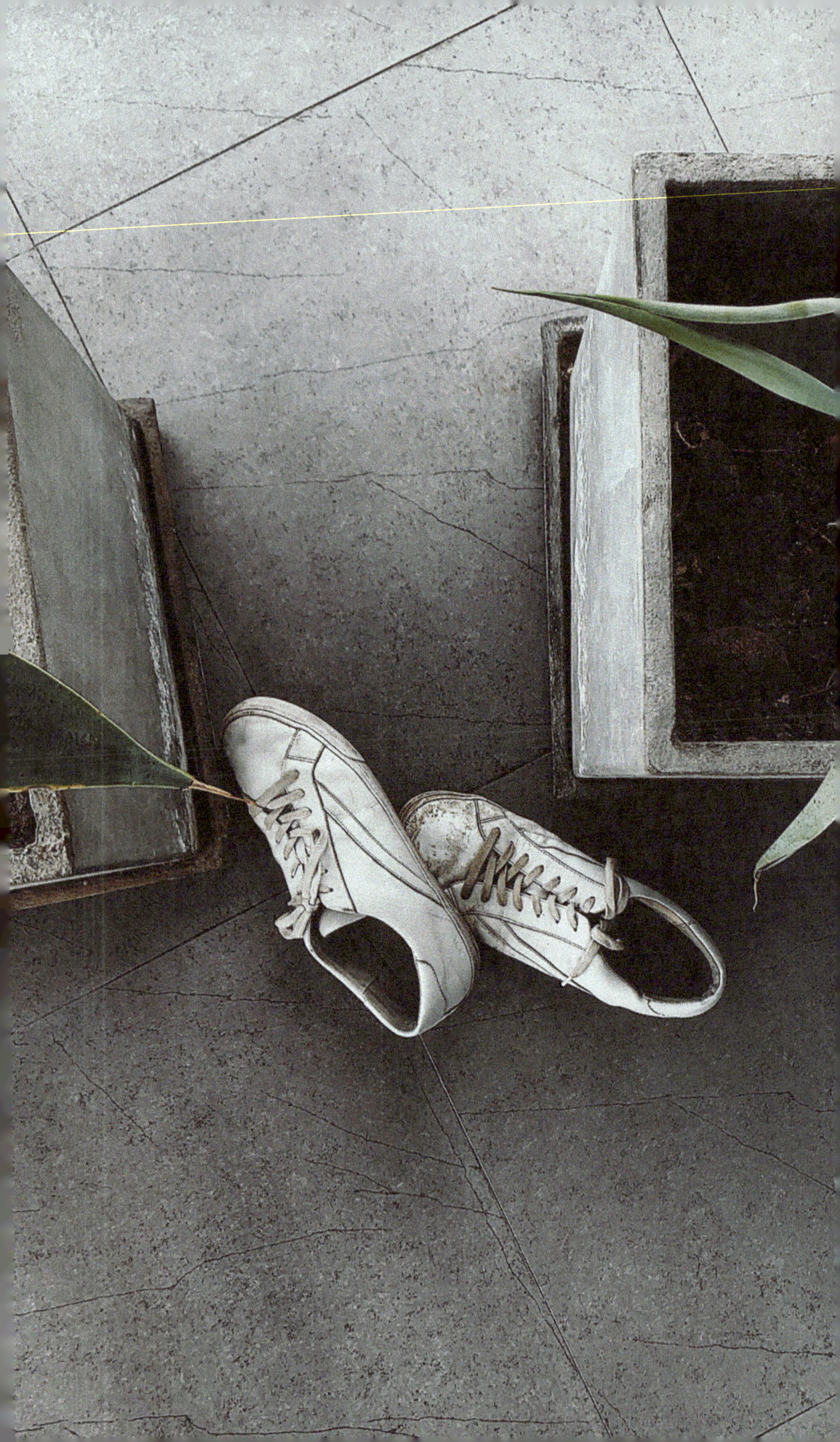

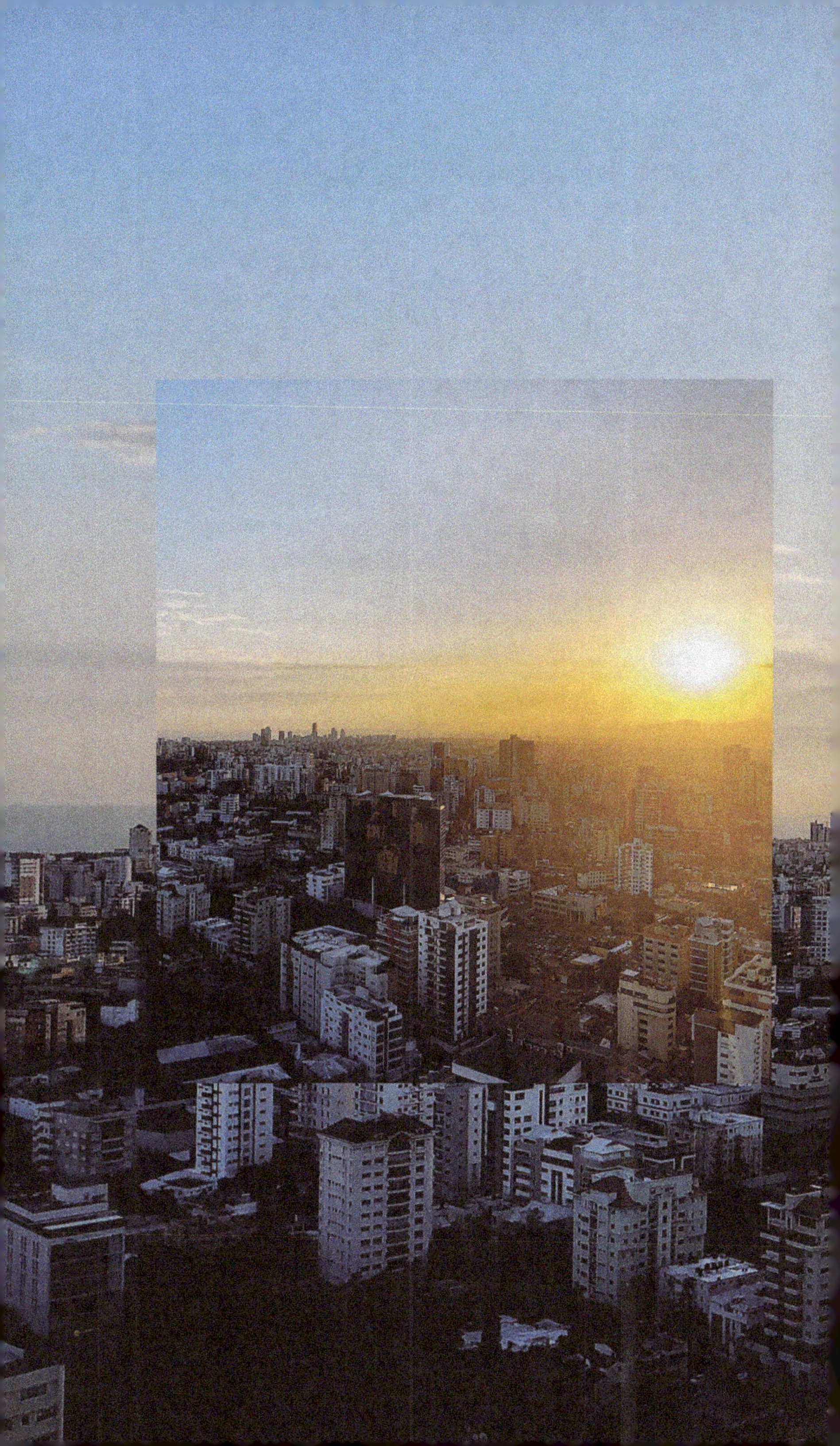

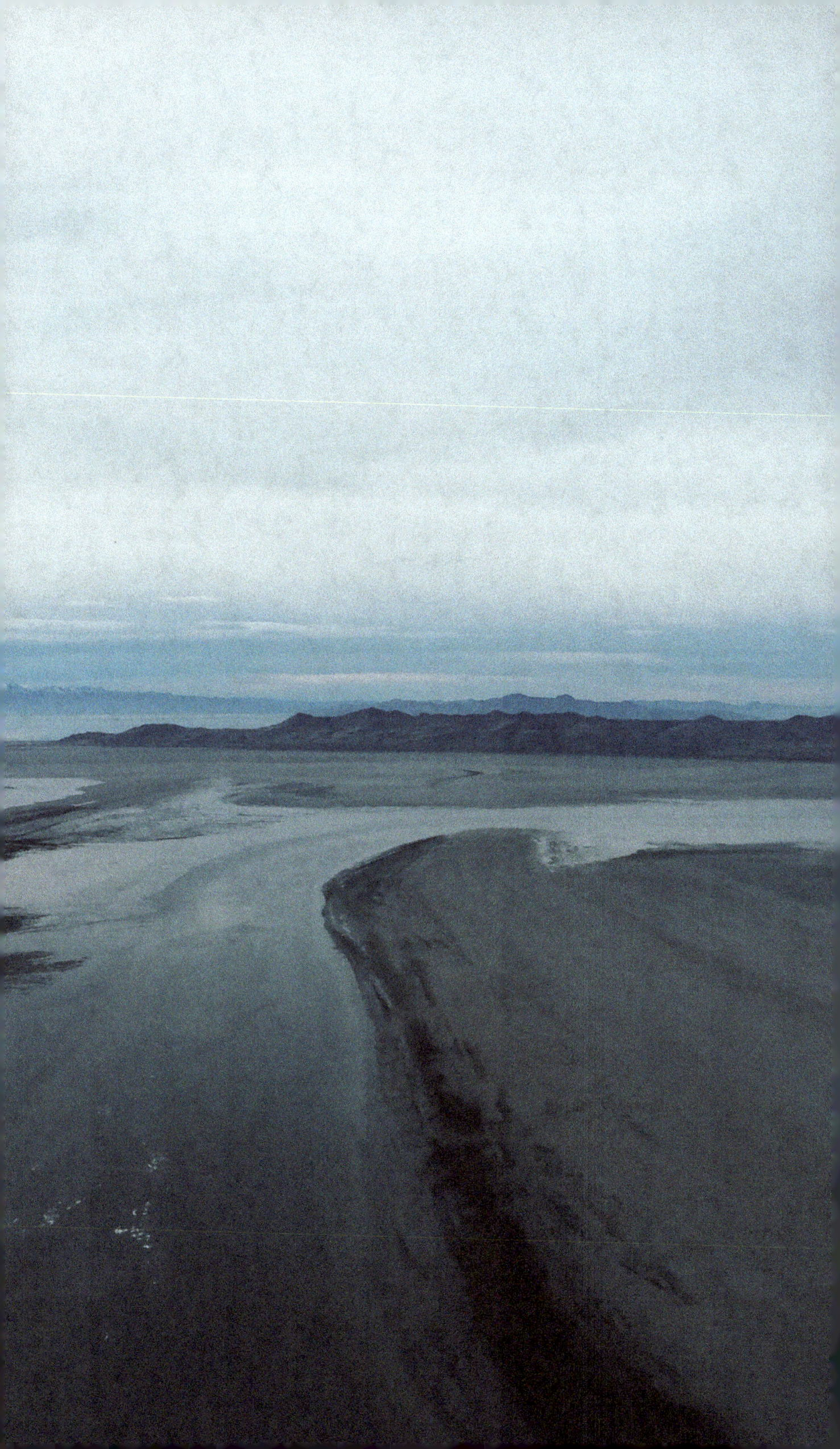

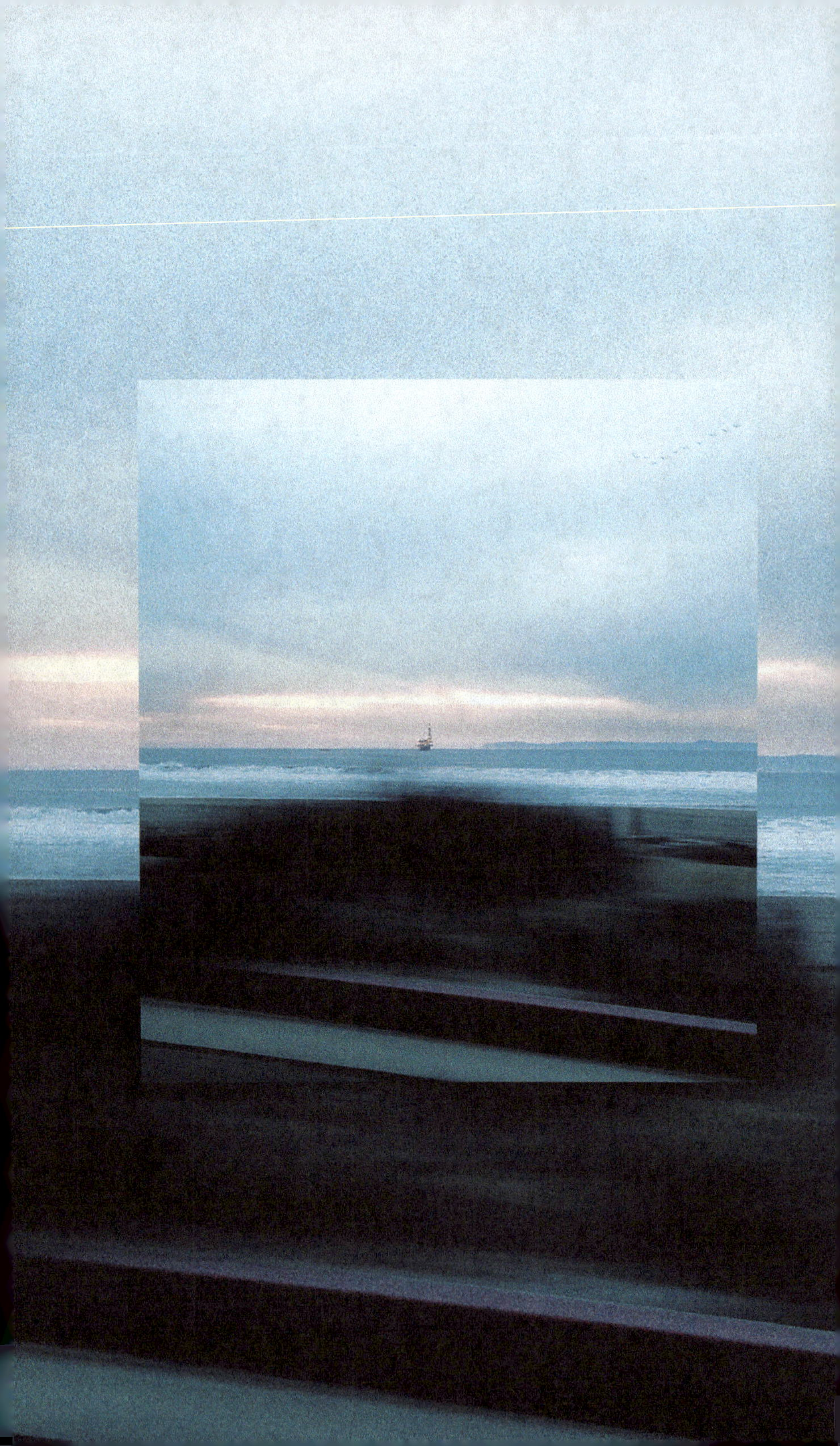

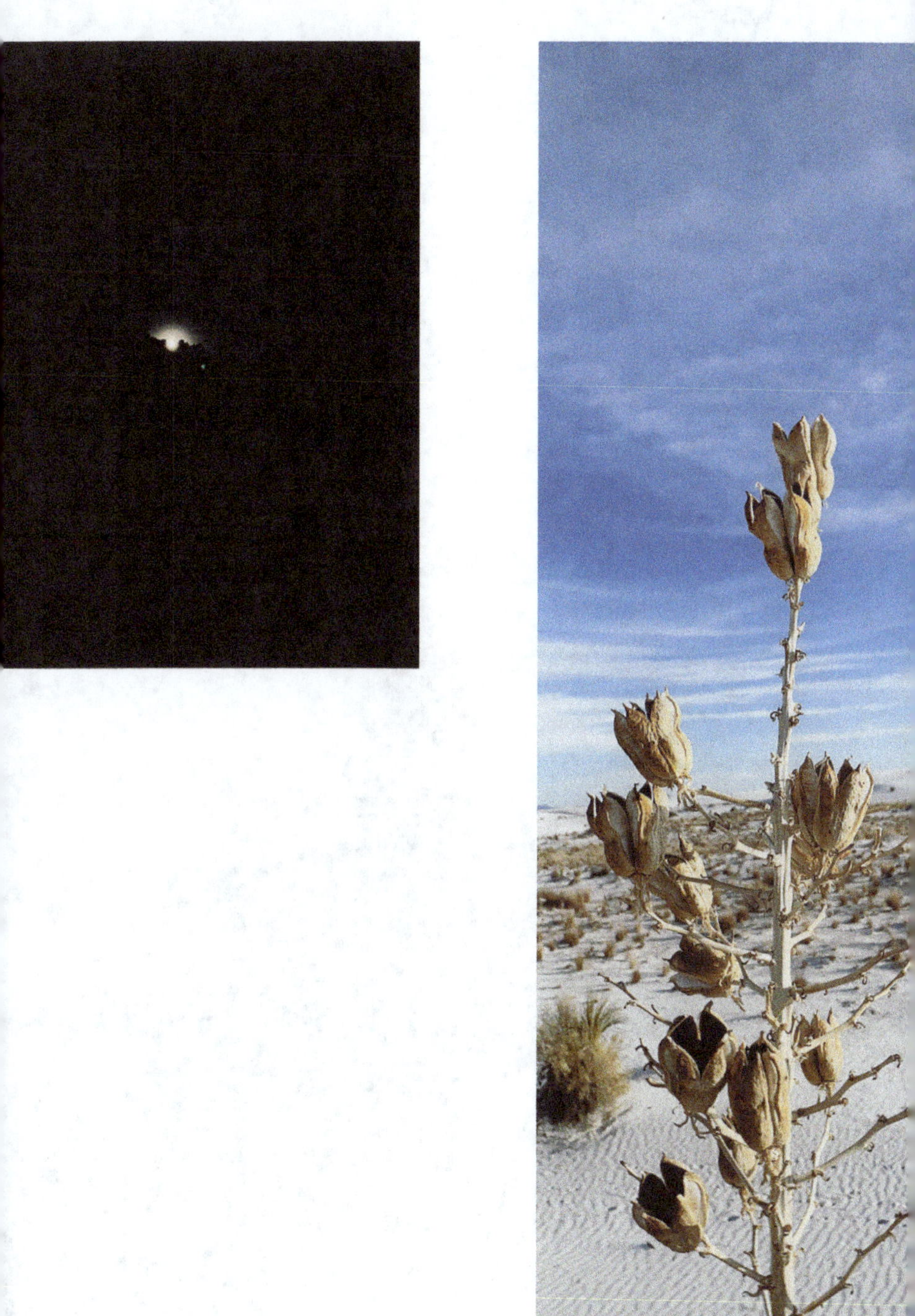

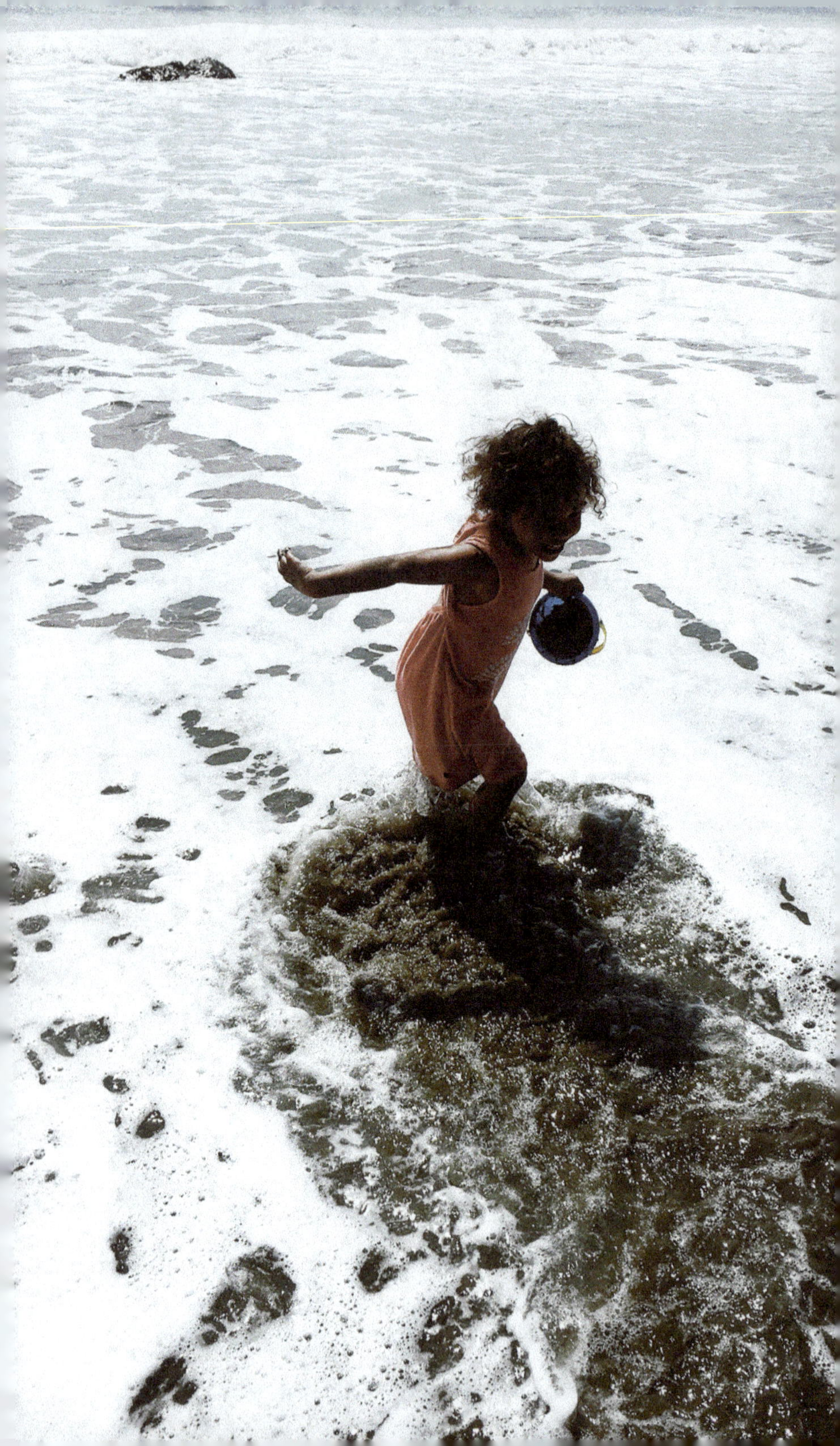

CHAPTER TWELVE

The Mastery of Habits

Our final principle is to take our prior three principles of *The Maguire Method* and shape them into a habitual routine. This is the most critical component of leveling up and ultimately transforming your life. This final principle is also the most difficult to implement. You see, we value our mental processing resources, so we are always trying to find easier ways to navigate around our world. We only have a limited amount of willpower to make decisions before it runs out.

Our brains often become tired and overwhelmed. As a result, most of our daily lives are made up of the same habits. We practice specific actions repeatedly, like brushing our teeth or locking our front door. This is why it's so challenging to reinforce our new actions. To do something out of the ordinary and expend additional effort without an immediate benefit actually takes up A LOT of our willpower. This is why you're too tired, bored, or busy to head off to the gym when you could just as easily turn an area of your home into a workout area.

When you're applying new habits to your life, it's so challenging to accomplish because it takes more time than what you would typically prefer before you see the results you're looking for. The longer timeline can be deflating if you're looking for immediate results and the reward you're seeking increasingly seems unattainable. So, we more often than not simply choose the path of least resistance.

It just takes time. So, how much time does it take to form a habit exactly? Does it take 21 days? Or is it 45? 66? Which is it?! If you've heard "21 days", you're not alone. This idea can be traced back to a book published in 1960 by Dr. Maxwell Maltz called *Psycho-Cybernetics*. Maltz referenced "21 days" as an observable metric in both himself and his patients at the time. He wrote: "These, and many other commonly observed phenomena, tend to show that it requires a minimum of about 21 days for an old mental image to dissolve and a new one to gel." His book became more popular (more than 30 million copies have been sold), so a situational observation became accepted as fact.

The truth is, it can take anywhere from 18 to 254 days for a person to form a new habit. It can take an average of 66 days for a new behavior to become automatic. There's no one-size-fits-all for this, which is why this time frame is so broad. Some habits are more accessible to form than others. Even more, some people may find it easier to develop new behaviors. There's no right or wrong timeline to creating a new habit. The only timeline that matters is the one that works best for you. For me, I found a sweet spot of 45 days to make the principles and steps I outlined in this book to become a habitual part of my daily routine.

A published study in the *British Journal of General Practice* states that habits are "Actions that are triggered automatically in response to contextual cues that have been associated with their performance." For example, you automatically put on your seat belt when you get into your car. You don't think about doing it or why you do it. Your brain likes habits because they're efficient.

When you automate actions, you free up mental resources for other tasks.

If we apply these tactics to actionable steps for our daily routines, no matter how small or large they are, one can deduce that we will have massive success. This is one of the reasons why this is the last but most crucial principle of *The Maguire Method*. If you repeatedly apply the previous principles, then you will get into a rhythm of creating a healthy and habitual daily ritual to get what you desire.

There is a unique tactic that you can try by gamifying your habitual routine by applying your practices and keeping records and scores if, like a game, it's much funnier to see the progress. For example, I found a lot of success by applying 30-day challenges to myself every month. Every month I would lay out a challenge of three goals for myself. One goal is career-based, one is personal, and one goal is a fun reward for myself.

My career goal might be to create a unique project with my team. A personal goal might be to teach my daughter how to play softball. My fun reward can be a weekend trip to Hawaii. I always made sure one goal was a stretch goal that I may not be able to conceivably achieve. However, if there is a will, there's a way. Then I have two short-term goals.

These goals may or may not fit into my overall long-term goals. It doesn't matter which one of the three is which. By the end of each month, I would keep track of whatever was accomplished, and whatever wasn't completed, I would add it to the next month. If all of my goals were achieved, I would create a new batch of goals. Because I made this into a game and something I set aside time for, it became a part of my habitual routine.

Thus creating a monthly 30-day goal-oriented challenge

became a habit. This began a snowball effect of achieving consistency, growth, and success (outward and inward). It always seems to be the most prominent concern people bring up when you challenge them to reach their goals and dreams. As we learned, that's not necessarily the absolute truth. There's more to it than that.

Yet we still yearn for that trick, hack, shortcut, or magic bullet that can give us more time. It's why a specific metric or number of hours we spend on something sounds so appealing. Like the 10,000-hour rule, best made famous by Malcolm Gladwell in his best-selling book, *Outliers*, Gladwell contends that 10,000 hours of "deliberate practice" are needed to become world-class in any field. He further writes that early access to 10,000 hours of practice allowed the Beatles to become the greatest band in history (thanks to playing all-night shows in Hamburg) and Bill Gates to become one of the richest dudes around (thanks to using a computer since his teen years). His theory is that once you've consistently put in that amount of time, the thing you're focusing on becomes a part of your lifestyle. It becomes secondary in nature.

However, this theory has been debunked countless times, as studies have found that practice does indeed matter for performance. But not nearly as much as the 10,000 rule suggests. The rule works differently for everyone. The secret to becoming a master of time and forming a successful habit lies in one thing… repetition. Repeating a behavior in the same context again and again.

It happens when we buckle up our seat belts in a car, log into our favorite social media channel when we're bored, or roam around in our fridge even though we're not really hungry. Repetition strengthens the connection in our brains between cues and the associated behavior. With enough repetition, our habits move from being initially conscious behavior to unconscious habits. So how do we create a new habit? It's the similar way we learn how to drive a car.

When you're driving for the first time, we are very conscious about every step we take and remember to shift gears while navigating our vehicle. Yet, over time and with repetition, we no longer use our conscious brain to drive ourselves to familiar places. The brain loves hardwire thinking but has a limited capacity to do so. We can only manage to change one habit at a time. This is why we can talk on the phone and drive once we have mastered driving (assuming that you are using a hands-free device, of course).

If we're able to use time management to our advantage, we should be able to build new skills and habits with repetition over time. I've applied this theory to my own lifestyle since I was around 12 years old. Since my family and I moved around so much, there was always a new time zone and culture to which I had to get accustomed. Time was always something I paid close attention to. My one constant was that I had an evening reward of watching primetime television.

So, more often than not, I would block my time around my reward. I would write out blocks of time on notecards to do my required tasks and hobbies I enjoyed. This allowed me to do something that is now commonly referred to as "time chunking". As I got older, this practice evolved but never stopped. I did everything from doing a different activity or task every hour on the dot to experimenting with two-hour blocks to even 15-20 minutes.

Because I never stopped this practice, time chunking became a part of my habitual routine. I can reveal to you what the results were from a firsthand experience. Firstly, this practice allowed me to be much more focused and efficient with the time that was presented to me. This allowed me more freedom to be flexible with how I spend my time. I also learned more about my body and temperament at different parts of the day.

This allowed me to schedule according to my own behavioral routine. I also learned that when you are intentional with what you do with your time, that fills your life with more substance. It's typically when we are unsure what to do with our time that our purpose isn't necessarily being fulfilled. Boredom can set in. Soon after, if not checked, so can depression, insecurities, and ugly little thoughts floating around in our minds come to the surface.

When we own the power of crafting a schedule that allows us more opportunities to get into a habitual groove, it gives us the space to design the life we always wanted for ourselves. Yet, even with that said, I also made time just to be bored and do nothing. Because that time was intentional, I found that a lot of creativity and thoughtfulness came during that time. So I was still safe-guarding my mental health.

Remember that there are 365 days in a year. This means that you have 365 opportunities. 365 chances to fail and succeed. That's plenty enough time to craft a routine that works best for you. 365 chances to take it one day at a time. One step at a time.

Imagine if you spent just 20 minutes of your day, every day or hell, even just some days working on a dream of yours. Do you know how far that will take you? It's time to create the world you always envisioned for yourself. Make that time intentional. Master your own habits.

CHAPTER THIRTEEN

We Live in a World of Ghosts

If we understand that forming a habit is critical to our success and that's common knowledge, why is it so difficult to do? For years, self-help books have sold millions upon millions of copies worldwide to provide you with actionable steps to improve your life. Yet self-help never goes out of style. Why is that?

One of the most famous names in the self-help world is motivational speaker Tony Robbins has once answered this very question in a podcast interview. The interviewer asked Tony why his business thrives even though he gives out the secrets of success and happiness. His response was very thoughtful and straightforward. He said most of the people that study his teachings and discover his lessons and advice don't actually apply them to their lives. He followed up by saying it's due mainly to people's inability to take the action they need to improve their lives because they get something out of their limiting beliefs that don't allow them to break free.

It is fascinating to know that we live in a world now where every single question that we might have, there lies some sort of answer out there somewhere for us. Even readily available and accessible. There is literally something for everyone. That's kind of the issue, isn't it? We live in a culture of instant gratification. This is a crucial reason why there is such a lack of effort and follow through with our growth and development as a species.

In fact, it is such a big problem that if something were not to happen as you desire fast and easy, then it appears as if you are doing something terribly wrong. From finding love, landing the perfect job, winning an argument, and making a ton of money to being on an undefeated streak of happiness whenever you want. If this isn't happening, what gives? Self-doubt, anxiety, an overwhelming amount of information, and continuously comparing ourselves to one another only makes this sting even more.

You have to do extraordinary things to get extraordinary results. Yet, so many of us are on the hunt for a magic bullet, secret trick, hack, tip, or fast track process to avoid entirely what is meant to be a rewarding process. When we intentionally try to avoid the process, more often than not, we will come up empty. When I think of this, the art of "ghosting" comes to mind for some reason. "Ghosting" is best defined as the practice of ceasing all communication and contact with a partner, friend, or similar individual without any apparent warning or justification.

Ghosting is followed by subsequently ignoring any attempts to reach out or acknowledge communication made by said partner, friend, or individual. This term originated in the early 2000s and became increasingly popular by 2015. Since then, ghosting has evolved. It can now happen between friends and family members and be practiced by employers with prospective candidates (and quite the other way around). In some ways, ghosting has been overused. This is especially the case in situations where someone goes on just one date with someone or meets someone once in real life, only to never hear anything from that person ever again. Our expectations are all over the place.

Ghosting may be especially harmful to those on the receiving end, causing feelings of ostracism and rejection. Some mental health professionals consider ghosting to be a passive-aggressive form of emotional abuse. It can be viewed as a type of silent treatment or stonewalling behavior and emotional cruelty. One could argue that ghosting is as apparent as any other form of rejection. The reason why it continues to be such a hot topic isn't just because it presents a different outcome than what we want from a situation.

It also highlights a trend of entitlement and lack of communication that's causing us to directly conflict with ourselves and our surroundings. However, the real issue with ghosting is the inherent ambiguity in ghosting in general. The person being ghosted does not know whether they are being rejected for something they or somebody else did. Those ghosted aren't even sure whether the person doing it is ashamed or they're scared of hurting the other's feelings. It may become impossible to tell which it is, making it even more stressful and painful.

Why do people "ghost" in the first place? There are various theories out there, but it boils down to this… the relative anonymity and isolation in modern-day living simply make it easier to sever contact with few social repercussions. In addition, the more commonplace the behavior becomes, the more we have become desensitized to it. Some even think ghosting is due to the decline of empathy in society, along with the promotion of a more selfish, narcissistic culture. I think all of the above is correct.

The strangest part about ghosting is how counterproductive it is. Since so many of us have been hurt by ghosting, and there have been multiple discussions about how it affects us negatively, you would think there would be *less* instead of more. Unfortunately, that's not the case. I've been the ghost, and I've also been the ghosted.

I faced one situation where I wanted to avoid ghosting altogether and just own up to softly bowing out of a romantic relationship that had gone on much longer than I wanted. It happened at a time when I didn't utilize any of the strategies shared in this book. It's also a great example of how lack of communication and the inability to use healthy habits can impact us negatively.

I had been dating someone for a few weeks. As it evolved, I understood it was a romance not meant to last. We had nothing in common, and it was during the season of 2020 when this relationship was more out of convenience than actual attraction. When she texted, I took my time responding. When she called, sometimes I picked up. Sometimes I didn't. The situation really took a turn during the Thanksgiving 2020 holiday.

We were still only a few weeks into dating, but I understood she wanted to spend the holiday with me. At the time, Covid-19 was all the rage. We lived in Los Angeles, and she couldn't visit her family in the Midwest. So essentially, she had no one to spend Thanksgiving with. She assumed I wouldn't have plans either.

But, I did make plans with my immediate family and scheduled a zoom video chat with my extended family to follow. I asked myself how I could handle the situation responsibly. After all, how could I live with myself if I ghosted this person on Thanksgiving? After giving it much thought, I asked her if we could go hiking the next day after Thanksgiving.

I thought maybe that would be an opportunity to see if there was a spark between us I didn't see before. If that wasn't going to be the case, I could at least break things off in person but be gentle about it. She agreed to my request. One of the main issues I encountered in this situation was that she overstepped her boundaries and frequently drank heavily. Because it was so early on in our relationship, I couldn't tell if this was just who she was or if she was dealing with the daily stress of the new world we lived in.

The holiday itself was chaotic. I was fielding *Happy Thanksgiving* texts and calls from family and friends to help prepare a meal with my family. My daughter was so pumped about the holiday she was practically bouncing off the walls.

The girl I was dating kept sending me text updates throughout the day too. I was just too busy to answer promptly or at all. All of it was just so exhausting that it made me want to ignore my phone altogether. I just wanted to get some sleep. So when my family left, that's precisely what I aimed to do after tidying up my place.

I remember finally collapsing on my bed and letting out a loud sigh of relief. At that exact moment, my phone rang, and I sent the call to voicemail. It was the girl I was dating. I told myself I'd call her back in a minute. Then she called again. Hung up. Then called again. Then a series of texts rolled in… *Why are you avoiding me?*, *Pick up, please, you're always ignoring me.* All of this happened within the span of just a couple of minutes. I stared at my phone in complete disbelief.

What the fuck was happening? Right then and there, I knew I had to part ways with this person. This would be the point in the story where I thought of simply blocking and ghosting her. After all, I was too tired to deal with any of this nonsense anyway. Instead, I texted her back, "I'll call you in 15 minutes." Then she called again and again.

This time I answered. As soon as I picked up, she laid into me, accusing me of avoiding her and not liking her. Before I could even respond, she started crying hysterically, explaining how lonely she was. I just patiently listened. I could empathize with her.

I had it pretty easy in comparison to her, spending time with my own family. I wasn't at all alone. It made perfect sense why she was so upset. I calmed her down. It was challenging because it became abundantly clear that she was drunk. So, I told her the truth. I told her how my day was, what I was doing, and that I didn't think it would be a great idea to continue seeing each other romantically.

She apologized profusely. She even added that she wasn't acting like her usual self. She cried again. She asked if she could just come over to hang out for a little bit. Against my better judgment, I said she could.

Huge mistake. She texted me the entire 20 minutes it took to get to my place in her Uber. When she arrived, her Uber driver called me. He told me that she wasn't in good shape and that he was concerned about her well-being. I immediately rushed outside to meet her.

I found her wandering in the middle of the street outside my house, crying. The Uber driver was standing outside his car, glaring at me. He gave me the "What did you do to her?" look. I had a "What the fuck is happening?" look. When she saw me, her face lit up. She collapsed in my arms, very loud and very drunk.

The Uber driver reluctantly left, giving me the eye the entire time. I brought her inside and poured her a glass of water. She was buzzing with adrenaline, pacing back and forth in my kitchen. Her sweater was stained with red wine. Her eye makeup was running down her face from her tears.

In between gulps of water, she went from trying to play Twista on her Spotify to wanting to watch a movie with me to demanding more bottles of wine to drink. Don't ask me why, but the Twista thing was my final straw. Finally, I told her that I was going to bed. She could sleep in my bed. I'd sleep on my couch.

She became distraught at the idea of not sleeping together. She reiterated she would leave me alone. She just didn't want to be alone. Once in bed, of course, she drunkenly tried to have sex. I refused. We spent the entire sleepless night tossing and turning.

The following day, she was a completely different person and acted as if nothing had happened. I did not. I wished her good luck with life and a brief goodbye after a shared cup of tea. Astonishingly, she texted me hours later, *I saw a cafe where we could have lunch and thought of asking you to come with me, but I realized everything is still closed.* I responded, making it abundantly clear that although she's a fantastic person, we were not a good match.

She replied, *Sounds good.* The End. Now. I know some of you are like, *See... that's why you fucking ghost someone. That's too much.* I disagree. The situation went off the rails because I was a poor communicator. If I had done that in the first place, then the problem never would have escalated and gone on as long as it did. Secondly, imagine if I did just ghost her.

Who knows how awful that would have made her feel. That would have been selfish of me. Ghosting is not a solution. It's a cop-out. It's avoiding an issue head-on because it's inconvenient.

Avoidance is a symptom of fear and those personal emotional wounds I mentioned before. Avoiding issues and not becoming self-aware can impact your life in ways you don't clearly see until it's too late. How we do one thing is how we do everything. While ghosting instead of having open communication may be easier and more convenient, it doesn't prepare us for other areas in life when we will need to show up and communicate.

From negative patterns to health issues, you make yourself a victim and become powerless in your own reality. When you take the time to face things head-on, that is true liberation and empowerment. It's an excellent opportunity for you and the other person to grow. How can we stop doing ugly habits like ghosting? Or drinking?

Or drug abuse? Biting our nails? Doom-scrolling? Overthinking things? How can we turn a bad habit into a good one?

According to Dr. Nora Volkow, director of the NIH's National Institute on Drug Abuse, the first step is to become more aware of your habits, so you can develop strategies to change them. One approach, Volkow suggests, is to identify the places, people, or activities that are linked in your mind to certain habits and then change your behavior toward those.

For example, if you have a substance use disorder, you can be deliberate about avoiding situations where you'd be more likely to be around the substance. This can help you achieve your goal of abstaining from using that substance. Another strategy is to replace a bad habit with a good one. For example, consider getting unsalted, unbuttered popcorn instead of snacking on potato chips. Instead of reaching for a cigarette, consider trying chewing gum or a flavored hard candy.

All of this will take time. If every day there is a little bit of progress, that's great. That's the whole point. This is a process.

CHAPTER FOURTEEN

Community: The Good vs. The Bad

If you want to reinforce your habits, you cannot do it alone. You will undoubtedly need support. As we've learned in countless examples, having a strong community and support system is critical to your success. Creating your own inner circle can also give you a healthier and fulfilled life. Since, for so many of us our online relationships are just as important as our offline ones, we should be exploring ways to nurture both.

In fact, Moira Burke of Carnegie Mellon University conducted a study that shared such insights. She found that interacting online with people you are close to by sharing messages, posts, and reminiscing about the past are linked to improvements in both personal well-being and strengthening offline relationships. She reports that "Staying in touch with these friends and loved ones brings us joy and strengthens our sense of community."

You should be mindful of allowing space for positivity and kindly excuse the toxicity out of your reach. This, unfortunately, depends on your background, including your family and certain friends. Whether that be an overbearing mother, a judgmental best friend, or a frenemy. Maybe you have trouble connecting and getting along with anyone for too long, or perhaps you do a great job of getting along with everyone.

The thing about self-help formulas is that they work wonderfully when you apply the new tactics privately. It becomes a different story when you have to apply them in real-world scenarios. Peer pressure, keeping up with the Joneses, and FOMO are real things. Let's not pretend that they are not.

Jim Rohn famously said, "We are the average of the five people we spend the most time with." If that theory is true, let's put it to the test with an exercise by creating what I referred to before as my "Impact List". First thing, make a note of the top 5 people you engage with the most. Put a {*} next to their names. Then jot down what you gain from that particular relationship and what you're contributing to nurturing it. Next, note the role that they play in your life.

Is it someone you look up to? Is it someone you see as your equal? Or is it someone you're looking out for? Next to their names, note this by annotating a "+" someone that is greater than you, "-" someone you can mentor, and "=".

Secondly, make a separate list of all the people you encounter daily, excluding strangers or chance meetings. If you're in a situation where you really don't interact with a lot of people but have a shit ton of online friends, that works too. Just make a list of everybody that's in your daily interactions.

Once you've done this, explore both lists and highlight everyone on your list that makes you feel good and empowered. Scratch out the names that make you feel uncomfortable and like complete shit. I want you to write a "?" next to the names of the people that you're unsure about how you feel about them. Take a step back and see what you've come up with. Think about it for a bit.

Craft a clear picture of how you impact others and how they impact you. You should come back to the list that you made for yourself from time to time and update it as you grow as a person. Some roles people play now in your life will eventually change. Some people will only be in your life for a season. That's okay. Appreciate the people you have in your life while they're here.

We live in a world where depression is at an all-time high as some of us are suffering in ways that we don't feel comfortable sharing in any sort of space. Some of us don't even know how much someone else might enjoy that phone call, text, or invite at all. Make sure that you do at least one thing to show love and empathy towards someone that's a positive presence in your life every day. Always be proactive about creating your inner circle and nurturing mutual support. At first, this may feel strange, but you will see extraordinary results.

I struggle at times to keep a consistent dialogue with my immediate family. We live in different parts of the country, and there's just so much we miss out on with each other's lives. So, I decided to be more proactive and start hosting family video chats. Everyone seemed excited for our first one. Then when the time finally came, they all bailed.

At first, I was hurt by this. It actually triggered a lot of self-limiting beliefs. It later dawned on me that this really wasn't our thing. Even when we're all together, we like to keep to ourselves. Instead of bowing out, I tried again.

The next time, everyone showed up. My family was excited to keep it going. Together, we were breaking generational curses and self-limiting behaviors by creating more opportunities for us to come together as a family. But maybe you're like me, where you are the one who always has to take the lead or make the first move.

It's something I've heard often from people as a deterrent to even bother nurturing their relationships.

Why should we put in all the work when someone else doesn't? The truth is that it's complicated. When you implement the principles, steps, and exercises we're exploring in this book, you will discover that you're not necessarily putting in all the work. You might just have a character trait that takes on more of the lead in some of your relationships. In that case, others know that about you.

This is why it's so vital that you know more about yourself first and then how that impacts your community. Now, if it's a one-sided relationship from which you gain nothing, then, of course, it would seem like you're putting in all the work. Those are the types of relationships that you discovered you can take away your attention and time from. They're draining and unnecessary. But, let's be clear, even nurturing relationships does take work.

But if you're getting the results you're seeking, then investing in relationships should be clearly worth it. Especially when you're reshaping dynamics and strengthening bonds. The energy you push out will always return to you. It's also okay to share your feelings with others if you feel like you're taking the lead in your relationships too much.

I have some family and friends who like doing specific activities together. Some enjoy sharing what they're working on with me. Others just love to laugh and exchange wild stories. It's different depending on each person. I make a note of that.

There are just so many different ways you can nurture your relationships. It can be as simple as sharing a funny meme or video, news article, or nostalgic memory. It can be even more thoughtful, like a mental health "check-in" message or sharing your gratitude for their presence in your life. Make time to hang out in person and do an activity you can bond over. Explore more ways on how you can show your support to them.

A few ways to do that are to exchange tips and advice on how you can level up your lives personally and professionally to reach your ultimate goals. You don't have to find any particular reason to deepen your bonds with people you care about. No reason at all is just as good. Always be open to different ways and styles of communication. Remember that any kind gesture is a good one.

Moving forward, create more opportunities to spend quality time with the people that empower you. Find ways to nurture your relationships with them. Spend less time with the ones that don't. Frequently, people find satisfaction in cutting ties with someone in a final conflict. You do not need to ignore anyone or shut them out of your life.

You can simply ease your foot off the gas and create space to focus on more of what and who you want in life. You're merely shifting your availability to be with healthier and positive influences in your life.

With the ones that you feel like you should distance yourself from, you have to be intentional about how you interact with them. Instead of hanging out every day, maybe it's every other day for "x" amount of time. What if it's someone you have to be around every day but don't like your interactions with? This applies to difficult coworkers, overbearing family members, toxic clingy friends, and your frenemies too. Find creative ways to limit your interactions with those people.

For example, I remember having to deal with an annoying co-worker. I made sure to give them ten minutes of my time each day. I even had a timer set to go off. When the timer eventually went off, I came up with a clever excuse to slip away. My whole point is to show you that you have way more of a say about who's in your life than you realize.

I've tried these boundaries myself and noticed how better my relationships have become. There's something funny about spending less time with people that makes you feel bad. They do notice. At the same time, you're consistently in such a better mood that it won't matter much. When I applied the exercise, I mentioned with a friendship I had, I loved the results. I discovered that this friend was quick to fuel drama, always asked for favors, and was quick to gossip.

The more I thought about it, the more I realized I didn't get much out of the relationship. When I pulled back on our friendship, not only did they notice, but they confronted me on it. They wondered if there was any beef between us. There wasn't. I was just investing my time in other opportunities. That's precisely what I said to that person.

I was happier to have space from that person and had no ill will towards them. Ironically, that person texted me asking for another favor right after that confrontation. I did not respond. They unfollowed me on Instagram the next day. People have a way of revealing themselves if you let them. I didn't even have to put in the effort of a confrontation. I let them confront themselves.

Nothing can stifle progress more than surrounding yourself with the wrong people. Some people in your life can be so damaging that they can pull you down and away from reaching your goals. As we learned, this is something that most people do unknowingly. In some relationships, whether they be professional or personal, they tear you down for what they think are benevolent reasons. They care about having you as they see you in their lives so much that they don't want to lose you to change.

When you challenge someone's reality and perspective, it's such a painful blow to their ego that they can respond in toxic ways (knowingly and unknowingly). Someone close to you that's witnessing you transform your life will have a tough time adjusting to the new you. In other ways, it's very true how the old saying goes, "hurt people, hurt people". Now, that's the most challenging part of creating successful habits. It isn't your unwillingness to put the work in. It's that you might be surrounded by one or more people in your life that can really deter you from getting the life you want for yourself.

You should feel comfortable setting firmer boundaries. Take a step back from relationships that weigh you down. Let's say you're having trouble spotting those red flags. A Journal of Consumer Research study found that friends often bond by providing one another with moral support to resist temptation. On the flip side, friends also can bond through common conspiracy to indulge.

Researchers discovered that when it comes to resisting temptations, like taking drugs or getting drunk, you and your friends are more likely to become partners in crime to indulge together than resist the temptations. You're likely to start acting like the people you surround yourself with too. If you surround yourself with people who make poor choices, you will get dragged down fast. If you choose those that inspire and challenge you to become better, you'll increase your chances of reaching your goals. You can discover who the type of people to surround yourself with by using our first principle of questions to ask if who's in your life right now is impacting your life in a positive or negative way.

You can then use the strategies laid out in our reflection principle to be sure they are in alignment with your own values. How can you determine who should and shouldn't be in your life? You need to recognize the healthy bunch from the toxic ones. Let's first take a look at the types of toxic traits you should be on the lookout for. Beware of these six types of toxic people:

1. **The Narcissist:** The Narcissist, can't help themselves from constantly interrupting you. They love to talk about themselves or just hear themselves speak in general. They don't ask you any questions. They don't wait for your responses either. They just won't shut the hell up in general.

   When they do, they're not really paying attention to you or anyone else. If something doesn't go their way, they're always victims. If something does go their way, it's because it's divine. In a relationship, these people will become completely self-centered and will never be attentive to your needs. They can be arrogant and see their own personal opinions as facts.

   This is because they often think they are the most intelligent person in the room, so they see every conversation and person as a challenge that must be won. They rarely see others as equals. This is why it's so challenging to try to form a connection with them. If you feel you are not being respected, step away while you still can.

   Narcissists are wired in a way that it takes some deep soul searching on their own part to discover the changes they need to make for themselves. Something to keep in mind, these days, we're too quick to label people narcissists when in reality, we all look out for ourselves first. It's human nature. A true narcissist sees you as a chess piece versus a human being, which shows in their actions. They see themselves as infallible.

2. **The Emotional Vampire:** This person sucks the air out of the room at any given moment. They bleed you dry of your positivity and leave you emotionally spent. They always have something sad, harmful, or pessimistic to say. Emotional vampires can never just see the positive side of things and tend to bring everyone down with them. These are the most dangerous types of people to have in your life because they can have you feeling defeated before you even get started with something you're passionate about. Even worse, they can take the wind out of your sails when you're really soaring. If you find yourself emotionally exhausted and feeling lower after hanging out with someone, chances are that person may be an emotional vampire.

3. **The Control Freak:** This person wants to control everything and everyone around them. Especially you. They want to be in charge of what everyone is doing, saying, and even thinking. If you disagree with them, they won't let the situation drop, trying to convince you that they are right. They rob you of your mental freedom, strip you of your identity, and drain you emotionally. This person will give you no breathing room and will wear you down until you are in complete agreement with them. If you are starting to feel like it's "their way or the highway" or are finding trouble being honest about what YOU want and your boundaries, I recommend creating some distance.

4. **The Liar:** This group includes liars, exaggerators, and the omitters of pertinent information… Whether they tell little falsehoods or major lies, it's exhausting to have a toxic deceiver in your life. Dishonesty drains us because we

constantly doubt their words, which can drive a wedge between our conscious brain and our own intuition. Having liars in your life can create an environment for gaslighting, making you question your own reality. That's terrifying. The presence of liars can truly make you go crazy and paranoid. If your intuition is telling you to watch your back, trust your gut.

5. **The Jealous Type:** Jealous people are incredibly toxic because they're experts at labeling you as the problem when, it's them. They have so much self-hate that they can't be happy for anyone around them. So they choose to judge, criticize, or gossip. According to them, everyone else is awful, uncool, or lacking in some way. If someone starts to gossip about other people to you, I'm here to tell you, they are 100% saying shit about you as well. This type can sneakily infiltrate your existence because they always add a bit of spice and excitement to things. In the long run, it does more damage to your psyche. Don't engage in their ways. Observe and then politely decline but never engage.

6. **The Drama Magnet:** Remember the story I told you about the self-saboteur? This is *that* person. Something is always wrong. Always. Of course, once a problem is solved, another one emerges. They're like chaos manifested. They only want your empathy, sympathy, and support. But not your advice. It doesn't matter that you want to help them and clearly see how they can solve their issues. Even if you offer help and solutions, they never seem like they want to fix anything. That's because they genuinely don't want to. Instead, they complain and complain. Their problems become more and more chaotic and unbelievable. Ironically,

they thrive in a crisis because it makes them feel important. So there is no real incentive for them to stop. They don't know any better. They're especially dangerous because the closer you are to them, the more drama they bring to your doorstep. You have been warned.

Now here's the thing. There are some great and even well-intentioned people that have toxic traits. You might discover that you may even identify with one or several of these categories. We all know someone that fits the bill with the above listed. But, no one can change themselves unless they genuinely want to for themselves. You can't force them to change.

However, if you make positive changes in your own life, others notice more often than not. They might even want to follow your lead. The best leaders lead by example, not by forcing someone to do what they think is best. Let's say you think it's best that you terminate some relationships (no matter how long and close they are to you). Maybe you're just on the fence about how to deal with someone in your life.

So, instead of being proactive about discovering a solution to dealing with them, you choose to do… nothing at all. You're not alone in this. You can be stuck at a job you hate for a lot longer than you should. You can be in a toxic relationship that you can't escape from. The key reason why most people struggle with letting go or even setting boundaries is guilt.

In order to free yourself from guilt, remind yourself that the happier and healthier you are, the more you spread positivity, inspiration, and love to someone else. That's infectious. In other words, finding your own happiness makes others around you feel happy too. If you're feeling the opposite, then the opposite effect is true. If you're conflicted about how you feel about someone, here are some great questions to ask yourself to determine how they make you feel:

- As I explained any of these toxic personality types, did someone pop into your head?
- Do you feel you have to constantly save this particular person and fix their problems for them?
- Do you get anxious and dread seeing them?
- Are you feeling drained after spending time with them?
- Do you get angry, sad, or depressed when you are around them?

If you discover someone in your life fits the bill, you should set boundaries and take a step back from the relationship. It's your life. You have to live it on your own terms. People may disagree with you, but they can't live for you. Only you can do that.

It has never been more difficult to set healthy boundaries than it is today. We live in a world where all of us have so much access to one another, in some cases without us even knowing. How can you effectively set healthy boundaries in the first place? Setting reasonable boundaries with someone professionally or personally speaking doesn't mean you can't also have a meaningful relationship with them. You don't have to wait until a line has been crossed before bringing up your boundaries.

Simply have a conversation with someone about both your boundaries. Introduce the topic gently by asking questions. For example, if you're in the beginning stages of dating, a great question to ask is, "What is important for you in your relationship?"

If they open up, that's an excellent opportunity to discuss your boundaries.

If not, then try again in a different way. Always notice what is essential for you and what boundaries you feel are being crossed. You can bring these up in other ways like, "When you do x, I feel y" rather than "It's horrible when you do x." If the person is reluctant to discuss boundaries, or if they react badly to you setting a boundary, this is typically a red flag.

In terms of dating, establishing boundaries is exceptionally daunting at first. When we're nervous about holding onto someone else's approval, we can compromise our own boundaries. Once you start doing that, your own sense of self can erode, and you can soon lose yourself in the relationship. If you don't know your own boundaries, pay attention to your instincts and your body. Typically we know when a boundary is overstepped because you're more likely to suddenly feel triggered emotionally within your body.

Setting boundaries in your personal relationships should be treated differently than setting boundaries in the workplace. The critical difference is that with our family and friends, it feels so natural to be able to talk about things like boundaries. Everyone has a better understanding since you know each other so well. However, at work, we often spend a lot of time with people we don't know as well or, even in some circumstances, people we haven't met in real life. What makes this even more complex is that our income and livelihood are tied so much to our work relationships.

We aren't always given the opportunity to discuss this in a way that feels natural for us. Just because it doesn't come naturally doesn't mean it's not something we should bring up and discuss together. Find a way to address someone without making the entire conversation about boundaries specifically. Lowering the stakes helps relieve some anxiety you may feel about what you need to discuss.

For example, suppose you have a one-on-one with your manager, and they reference an email or message that was sent after hours. In that case, you could say, "I've stopped checking my email in the evenings so that I can make sure I am taking time to rest and spend time with my family during off-hours." You can add on to that statement with a firm expectation of when you will respond and when you're next available to work on the given task. Saying "*no*" in the workplace or in life isn't easy. We're so consumed by the idea of taking on everything that we neglect how that truly impacts our overall happiness and productivity.

Getting comfortable with speaking up when your workload feels like it's piling on top of you is an excellent way to establish boundaries for yourself. I listed the toxic traits to watch out for first because I wanted you to have a more straightforward path about what you need to avoid. Now, here are seven character traits of people that you should embrace. If you know of anyone that fits any of these categories, make more space for them, and attempt to bring them into your inner circle:

1. **The Kind Heart:** This person is willing to offer you anything you need. From kind words to their network list to even some financial aid to help you pursue your dreams. The kind-hearted friend is generous and desires to see your progress. If they notice your potential, they genuinely feel they owe it to you to give you what you need to

be successful. Whenever you need them, this person has your back.

2. **The Optimist:** When you are overwhelmed with challenges and obstacles, you need this kind of person to help you see the positive angle from where you are. An optimistic view takes you in the right direction and enables you to focus on results rather than your limitations. This person wants you to know that everything will work out for your own good. The best ones work through your problems with you and then break them down enough so you can see a way out. This is critical to note. They help you find a solution that works for you. Not them.

3. **The Devil's Advocate:** This person looks at what you're doing logically and critically. They're great at identifying your game's weaknesses and keeping you grounded. Where an optimist says to look at the bright side of things. The Devil's Advocate prepares for potential dangers.

   Their truth stings like hell, but it's the hard truth you always need to hear. This is tricky because they can be confused with a toxic trait if you're not open or comfortable with constructive criticism. They're not here to create more obstacles for you or dissuade you. Instead, they offer you perspective and insight into how to improve a given situation. For example, this person does not say, "I don't think this idea is going to work. Sorry." or "Isn't someone else doing that too? Sounds like a waste of your time."

   Instead, they say, "I don't quite understand the idea. Have you thought about xxx or thought about xxx?", "Have you considered trying this?", "I would recommend you look out for xxx", or "You're usually more attracted to this type of person. But they always end up hurting you. Have you ever thought of dating someone like xxx?"

4. **The Mentor:** The mentor is someone who has experienced life in ways you haven't yet. They can give you a roadmap to help you on your journey. They certainly have made mistakes and have lessons from them which they can impart to you. They are concerned about your growth and are willing to provide you with advice, guidance, and perspective.

   Be mindful of who can be a mentor in your life. I get asked this often about how you can find a great mentor and what to look out for. It's not as difficult as you think. Find someone who has more experience than you do, a person of high value that you have respect for and ask them if they can guide you and impart their wisdom to you. Take the lead and set aside time to just chat with them regularly when they are available to do so.

5. **The Loyalist:** A.K.A. your "ride or die" or your "partner in crime". This is your companion, a buddy, or a full-time supporter of your cause. They have skills that you can learn from them. They are astute and make opportunities happen for the both of you. They are really effective because they know you like no other person does and have always been present in your life. They always want you to succeed. To them, you can do no wrong on this journey to reach your goals. They are there for you all the way, and they rarely retreat, even going to great lengths to help you succeed, even in the face of ridicule. They believe in you, your dreams, and will always be your loyal companion.

6. **The Visionary:** What separates this role from that of the mentor is that this inspirational figure could be more of the role model rather than someone who guides you through the hurdles of success. The inspirational figure can be more distant from you. They're solid in deeds and character, serving as the ideal model for you to follow.

7. **The Work Bud:** This person knows your struggles and the challenge of overcoming them because they're going through the same thing. It's a reciprocal relationship you need and will appreciate when your work-life gets tough. They can help you by covering the small stuff while you give the lion's share of your attention to your top priority at work. You'll find that you'll pick up the slack for one another at work when one of you needs to focus on your own top priorities (personal or professional). Perhaps the most significant benefit they provide is friendship and camaraderie. Having true friends at work makes us happier. When we're more content, we're more productive. When we're effective, we can get more done in a shorter amount of time, so it's easier to put the focus back on our personal life.

When you have a tight-knit squad of excellence, you're primed for happiness, fulfillment, and success. Strong-willed friends can increase your self-control. If you struggle to resist temptation, surrounding yourself with people who possess a high degree of self-discipline helps. Studies have shown that when people run low on self-control, they often seek out self-disciplined people to boost their willpower. Since self-control is so vital to reaching long-term goals, befriending people with the ability to do this is the secret to success. Especially if this particular group of people share your core values.

Whether you're tempted to skip that workout at the gym or you're considering blowing this month's budget, spending time with a disciplined friend boosts your motivation to maintain healthy habits. Pay attention to the company you keep, and be mindful.

We should also be mindful of how we manage our online relationships. While bonding over internet jokes or posts can strengthen your connection to someone, their social media content might also become a concern. Maybe someone posts something you disagree with, or someone you know in real life shares a different side of their personality online. Before confronting anyone, think about how the conversation would go in person.

Don't respond to a post or comment out of emotion. Focus on responding vs reacting. Take the time to process what you have read or seen. Always allow yourself the grace of time to reflect on your thoughts before commenting out of anger or frustration. While you may be tempted to share all aspects of your life online, don't. If it's something you wouldn't overshare with your loved ones, neighbors, colleagues, and extended acquaintances in real life, it probably shouldn't be on social media either.

However, you approach your life on the internet, be mindful to think about your relationships in person before online. Remember who your friends are. Before sharing your thoughts or posting something provocative or controversial, keep your audience in mind. Is it worth creating tension with your family, friends, or co-workers? Keep your personal conversations personal. There is nothing to be gained by taking your private life public.

As a public figure, I have learned this first hand by facing criticism from family members and friends by sharing some personal experiences publicly. So, why even risk alienating your loved ones or potentially harming your reputation? It's easier to just not, isn't it? When you do that too often, it confuses what your priorities really are. Does it matter more to post a photo of you on a summer beach vacation with a loved one or actually enjoying your summer beach vacation with a loved one?

This applies to romantic relationships too. The concept of finding love online is actually not as unlikely as it may sound due to instantaneous connections and the ability to scroll through someone's likes, dislikes, or favorite memes. It's pretty easy to find common interests with someone and to slide into their DM's to initiate a conversation. Some romantic relationships can begin through social media but can also be damaged by it. Whether it's liking someone's photo or your partner is talking to other people online, it's easy to become jealous of our partner's experiences online.

According to Leslie Shore, an interpersonal communications expert and author of *Listen to Succeed*, "Research shows that, on average, we spend two or more hours a day on social media. Those who have limited experience in reading people do not have the same level of social intelligence that previous generations possess. If this becomes the new normal, building strong, deep relationships will take more time and will be more difficult to maintain."

You don't need to put your phone down entirely. You don't need to delete your favorite apps either. Social media can be exciting, fun, and a great way to relax or keep up with people from afar. You just need to find your own healthy balance between both sides of the screen.

Healthy habits are hard to develop and require changing your mindset. But if you're willing to make sacrifices to better your life, you can clearly see the impact can be far-reaching, regardless of your age, sex, or physical ability.

CHAPTER FIFTEEN

You vs. You

A University of Scranton study in 1988 discovered that 77% of people who committed to a New Year's resolution only stuck to it for a week. Only 19% of those who made resolutions actually fulfilled them within two years. The statistics have only grown worse over time. Now, around 4% of people who made New Year's resolutions said they kept them. So, if you didn't stick to your New Year's resolutions, you're not alone.

If creating a brand-new habit in the first place is difficult, it's no wonder that evolving it into a routine and a way of life is nearly impossible for some people. For example, at the end of every year, most of us get excited about the prospects of a new year. After all, we can right the wrongs in the new year. We even get a chance to reflect on all of the things that we accomplished in the previous year with a newfound hope that what's to come is just around the corner. Every year begins with a brand new sense of energy that's infectious to everyone around us.

We turn this into a goal mindset. In most cases, this is great. If you're like me, you make a list of goals and try to attack each one. Yet somehow. Some way. It all fizzles out.

What typically happens is we just simply become complacent. Boredom and disinterest emerge if we don't see quick results. As we've learned, there are no immediate results in a process. Even though that makes sense, it's more often than not complex to believe that. So, when we don't see massive changes happen quickly from the new methods we're trying, we just give up.

The issue is that we're looking at the process with the wrong mindset. We're looking at our new habits through the lens of a goal-oriented mindset versus a growth mindset. You should have goals, but in order to get into the habit of achieving them more and facing challenges with a better head on your shoulder, you have to shift your mindset. You have to embrace a growth mindset.

Our worst enemy is usually ourselves. Most of the time, we don't even recognize that. Self-sabotage is the self-fulfilling prophecy of things going wrong. All of us do this. Most of us don't even know why. The causes are complicated as we humans are complicated. It can be easy to slip into the role of self-sabotage.

Sabotaging ourselves is rooted in fear and can come across in many different ways. It can look like blaming others when things go wrong or choosing to walk away from a situation when things don't go smoothly. It can be procrastination or picking fights with friends or partners, dating people who aren't right for you, communicating your own needs too quickly, or even putting yourself down. These types of behaviors can come from patterns we learned in childhood. These patterns lay down the groundwork for our perception of our early relationships.

Throughout life, we're attached to these repeated patterns, and that's what makes them so hard to move past. They become the type of habits that we have to break free from. You can also come from a past relationship dynamic where you didn't feel supported or heard. When you asked for what you needed in previous relationships, romantic or otherwise, you might struggle to communicate effectively in your current relationships.

Those recurring dynamics and the fear of the unknown prevents us from genuinely becoming successful at gaining what we want in life. You might ask yourself a series of questions that will cause you to overthink or slow you down even if you are making progress. If you get that new promotion, will your job put more pressure on you? Will you be able to rise to the occasion when the time comes? Will you know what to do?

This train of thought leads to self-defeat. All too often, we don't quite understand the strength of our subconscious mind and how the action that we take against ourselves is not premeditated or conscious at all. If you've ever been in an argument and you get angry, you typically say things you don't mean. It isn't because you're conscious of what you're saying. It's because you're not. The same thing could be said when it comes to self-sabotage.

I knew someone who referred to themselves as the "unluckiest person on the planet". But on the outside, looking in, she had it all. She's greatly desired and admired. She's intelligent, kind, resourceful, and always looking out for others. She's the type of person that can walk into a room and get anything she wants easily without saying a single word. Even when she failed at things, she failed up.

So why did she claim she was so unlucky? Well, she experienced childhood traumas. Traumas that were no fault of her own, but she accepted that narrative as a part of her identity. As she grew older, whenever she achieved her goals, it felt more like a happy accident than something she deserved. She would openly and consistently question her own abilities and choices.

This would happen even more when someone noted how easy

it appeared for her to manifest things. Quite simply, she didn't think that she deserved it. Imposter syndrome was a daily struggle for her and difficult to overcome no matter what she accomplished for herself. So, in response to this, she would put herself in chaotic romantic entanglements and procrastinate to the point of missing out on game-changing career opportunities. When things didn't work out, she boldly declared that she was just unlucky and had no idea why bad things happened to her.

One morning, she received an email invitation for her to speak on a prevalent platform where as fate would have it, was the exact pay she needed at the time. She was falling into debt and needed a big payday to help her out. When this opportunity came (seemingly out of nowhere), it was truly divine intervention. As she went on her drive to this speaking gig, she called me in a panic.

She was late to her speaking gig and no longer wanted to go. Hearing the panic in her voice, I attempted to talk her through things. She was driving at a peak traffic time on the 405 freeway in Los Angeles. I just wanted to make sure it was safe. I reminded her this was an excellent opportunity, and it wasn't anything she hadn't done before.

She settled a bit. As soon as I got off the phone with her, I had this unsettling feeling in the pit of my stomach. I could feel the energy of her anxiety seeping through our call. Only 10 minutes later, she would call me crying because she had gotten into a car accident.

Luckily, there were no serious injuries. But mere minutes after our chat, she plowed into another car on the freeway. She says she doesn't remember how it happened exactly. But because of her accident, she no longer had to attend the speaking engagement she was going to. Neither did she get the check she needed. She was gifted with the art of self-sabotage in a way that I've never quite seen before. Her car was totaled.

Afterward, I drove to her best friend's house. Upon hearing her version of events, her best friend laughed and replied, "Damn bitch. You're like the unluckiest person I ever knew". They both shared a laugh as I just stood there in this surreal moment. She obviously had no problem sharing her self-proclaimed label often.

It's hard enough to challenge our own self-limiting beliefs but to have rallying support behind it does more damage than good. Even if it's in a fun-loving way, it's harmful. In retrospect, she was great at dropping self-sabotage bombs all over the place. It was only a matter of time before something detonated. After a while, she set off a bomb of self-sabotage between us. When that happened, I gently pulled away and put my energy elsewhere.

It would be several months later before we reconnected. When we did, she had a completely different vibe about her. This time, my friend was very self-aware and made healthier lifestyle choices for herself. She owned her power now instead of owning the title of "the unluckiest person on the planet".

One day we spoke about her car accident in particular. Her face lit up when I brought it up. She told me she still doesn't quite remember what happened but what she said next was even more intriguing. She told me, "You know… there's a part of me that thinks I did that on purpose. I don't know. There was just so much going on at the time. It all felt very overwhelming."

I responded by sharing the theory I privately held about the situation. I thought she got into a car accident to continue her "unlucky" narrative. She told me she was relieved when she got into that car accident. She laughed, followed by a bit of retrospective honesty. It took the pressure off her to level up to a standard she wasn't yet ready to fully embrace.

As her story unfolded, she became more conscious of holding herself accountable for her actions instead of continuing on a destructive path. With the car accident in particular, maybe to her it was easier than facing the challenge of speaking onstage? After all, countless studies have shown that most people fear public speaking even more than death. One of the reasons why we sabotage ourselves even when it's working against our best interest is because we still get something out of it. You might feel unfulfilled at work because your daily tasks don't use any of your unique skills.

So, instead of figuring out what you could do about it, you'd rather avoid it altogether and hit happy hour hard every night after work. You might tell yourself you want to be in a serious romantic relationship even though you're the happiest when you're single. In response, you start creating conflict every time you move past the casual dating stage. Start understanding and identifying your behaviors. For example, maybe you detach from relationships and pick fights once your partner says, "I love you." Perhaps you have a pattern of quitting jobs right before your annual review.

Take the time to understand what truly sets you off. Which triggers you? Is it boredom? Fear? Or maybe even things are going too well for you? How about self-doubt? Track your triggers in a journal. Then use some of the steps outlined in our principles to help you gain sharper insights and non-judgment awareness.

If you notice specific patterns keep appearing in your life, seek more feedback from people you're close to. Let them show you yourself from a different perspective. This will help you break self-sabotaging behaviors by holding yourself more accountable.

Progress is non-linear. Sometimes you take two steps back, one step forward, or even five steps sideways. This is frustrating for even the most patient of us. Maybe you'll get bored. Perhaps you'll slip up and fail again, even more significantly than you ever have.

At the beginning of 2020, I hit milestones and overcame challenges with inspiring momentum. Many of the challenges and obstacles I mentioned in this book were behind me. I began the year toasting champagne on the sandy beaches of Peru with some of my best friends as fireworks lit up the night sky. I was Face Timing with my best friend and the love of my life. Business was good. Life was good.

I remember this feeling of being finished with many things that dogged me in the past. I was ready to go upward, and nothing could stop me. But that feeling was short-lived. Within one week, my aunt suddenly died, my basketball hero, Kobe Bryant, died tragically along with his daughter, and my crucial client, out of nowhere, decided to shake up their leadership, and I was on the chopping block. They didn't even want to honor our agreement and pay me the monies owed.

Then there was financial uncertainty once again. I panicked at the thought of going through what I had been through before. Then the final blow came from my romantic relationship ending suddenly.

Every day, something new and awful was happening to me. It didn't feel like it was for me. I tried many of the steps, strategies, and recommendations I outlined in this book. It was going according to plan until it wasn't. I wasn't even angry.

I was just confused. Shouldn't I have this fantastic comeback story or a tale of triumph over failure? What was I doing wrong? What was the universe trying to tell me?

Then I had a gentle self-reminder. It was up to me to figure this out on my own. It was up to me to respond the way I wanted to. I knew I didn't understand why so much chaos was happening, but I did understand no one was conspiring against me. So, I acted fast using *The Maguire Method* to shake things up and re-examine my identity.

I became re-energized. I understood this was my opportunity to show the universe what I got. I made so many plans. I was relentless with my career and personal pursuits. I was ready to fulfill my destiny and purpose.

The universe responded with my dedication and grit with opportunity after opportunity. I was in hot demand to publicly speak at popular venues around the globe especially at places listed on my bucket list. Bigger and larger partnership deals were filling my inbox. Contracts were signed for longer commitments. More money was on the way, and a roadmap of abundance became clear.

My entire year was being laid out in front of me in a way I had never experienced before. Then, everything came to a screeching halt. Yet again. COVID-19 emerged and ripped a fucking hole straight through any plan I had. Except for this time, it wasn't just me.

It was the entire world. There was nowhere to run or hide. Some of us couldn't even just push through. Most of us just had to... wait and think. Then wait some more.

Within hours, massive shutdowns and quarantines evaporated my plans into vapor. As more details emerged, panic and fear crept up inside me. My daughter and her mother were safe and nearby. But the rest of my family was on the other side of the nation. To top it off, the one person I confided in and talked to about all this chaos was no longer part of my life.

It didn't just feel like my entire world was falling apart. It felt like nothing mattered anymore. I slipped into bad habits. I began asking all of the wrong questions more and more. Even during my reflection periods, it didn't mean much.

After all, all I could do was think about things and how everything seemed to be turning into shit. Every action I took felt meaningless. Eventually, I realized there were more crucial life lessons I still needed to accept. So, I applied *The Maguire Method* principles… again. I asked different questions that challenged me to re-examine not just my purpose but how I showed up in the world around me.

When I reflected on the new answers that I found I soon discovered that no matter what was happening in the world around me I had to remain steady with my own integrity and my spirit. Then I took swift action even if some of that action meant being better about waiting and preparing. Even if I couldn't do all of the things I wanted or the way I wanted, I did what I could. If I couldn't go to the gym, I'd work out from home.

If I couldn't travel around the world to speak, I would instead speak from my home, and continue to plan what my traveling would look like when I could again. I simply chose to let go of things out of my control. Finally, I molded this way of thinking and action to fit my lifestyle choices. I created new habits. I took things one step at a time. I recognized the progress soon after.

As time went on, chaos erupted in the forms of polarizing politics, social justice, climate change, and more. Every day there was something new. For me, the spotlight on the Black Lives Matter movement was tension-filled. Strangers were less concerned about catching coronavirus as they were about coming up to me to share their views in support (or quite the opposite of) the movement. Every part of me now had to find a new way to not just thrive but survive in an environment that was increasingly becoming unpredictable.

The persistent voice inside of me only grew louder. I was made for these times. Every lesson learned. Every bit of pain. Every bit of success. Every bit of knowledge and wisdom. Every bit of love and support. I dedicated myself to being an unstoppable force and an immovable object.

I revisited every single philosophy I learned. I read countless journal passages. I had numerous conversations with people from my past, present, and new voices. All the while, I was continuing to change, learn and evolve. Some days were longer than others. Some days I felt like I was on top of the world. Other days, I felt small and insignificant.

Yet I continued. I survived anyway I could. As unemployment went to a record high and conspiracy theories became the norm, another challenge emerged. I couldn't rely on consistency any-more. After all, each day was becoming more erratic. Instead, I recognized inconsistency as its own pattern and got into a groove of how I could react to things outside of my control. No matter what, I just continued moving forward.

In retrospect, the coronavirus came at a time of uncertainty about where human civilization was and where it was going. The world itself decided we should be in "time out". It changed every-thing. Not just for me but all of us. You have stories of your own about how this moment in history impacted you.

So many of us went through our challenges and journeys during this time, from re-examining our work life to contemplating how we spent time with our loved ones. Hell, we even examined our own mortality and purpose on this planet. By now, you have realized it's entirely up to you how you respond to the world around you. How you want to feel about any situation is entirely up to you.

You get to decide if you want to take action any way you want to. The truth is that you have much more power than you're even aware of. You give up that power to other people or to other circumstances because you think you're powerless. You're not. You are powerful. Your life has meaning and purpose.

Even when you think you have it all figured out, life has a way of reminding you otherwise. Time and time again, when things don't go as we expected or planned, we can fall into the trap of thinking we did something wrong. Understand this. Nothing will ever go according to plan. Because whatever plan you had in mind was never designed to do that. Life is unpredictable, and we are all imperfect beings.

It doesn't matter how skilled you are, how privileged, or how many goals you achieve. You'll never be perfect. You will never have *it* all figured out. You will sometimes fail.

You will sometimes succeed. You must always continue moving forward. If you run a marathon, you might stumble. Even fall. You have to dust yourself off.

Always finish what you started. You might not even finish the way you envisioned. But you must continue to rise again and again until you do. The only wrong choice you can ever make is the one where you give up.

Never give up. Always keep going

Sunsets

My toes are in the sand again. Back where I started. I'm watching the sun get swallowed up by the darkness this time. Like I said before, this is a familiar place, but it doesn't quite feel the same. I know I mentioned in the beginning how I prefer sunrises to sunsets. However, that's not to be confused with me liking one and not the other.

They're one and the same. The beginning is the end. The end is the beginning. I should never have separated the two. After all, how can you recognize light without the dark? How can you be mesmerized by the glowing beauty of the world without experiencing its absence?

At this moment, I am breathing. I am smiling. I am full of joy. I am also not alone. My daughter is nearby, laughing and dancing in the sea. She splashes the water all around her. Her laughter is infectious. I hope she never stops smiling. I know there will be times when she will. I know she'll be disappointed and feel the pain of the world.

I also know that she will experience the beauty of it all too. She will indeed experience the sour, but she will also experience the sweet. If you are so lucky to have a child of your own, there are moments in life where you reflect on the life you lived that made you who you are. If I wouldn't have experienced so many of life's challenges, then I wouldn't be able to be a better man for her. If I never suffered, I never would have been able to empathize with you or pass on lessons learned. That makes me smile.

My story is still being written. Life's challenges never disappeared. In fact, they only became more complex. That's life. With *The Maguire Method* I was well-equipped to deal with those obstacles while enjoying the highs including the small moments I'm appreciating right now.

My daughter runs up to me excitedly. She must have caught my gaze. She's soaking wet, as free as one could be. She asks me to join her in the ocean. I kindly decline. She pauses for a moment before shouting, "I love you, daddy!" Within seconds she leaps back into the sea.

The sun's almost gone now. When it disappears, the darkness will come, but the shining sun will always return as it always has. That makes me think of scars. Our scars define us. For some of us, they are more significant than others, but all scars heal. Have you heard that before?

Our emotional scars are like open gushing wounds. Something happens if you leave it, ignore it, or pretend it's not there. It gets worse and becomes infected. It eventually consumes you. However, if you treat it with the proper attention, something else entirely happens.

When you take the time to discover the appropriate medicine needed, your wounds will heal if you take the necessary steps to heal yourself. You'll be surprised to learn you can also recover the other parts of yourself. It is true what they say. Hurt people, hurt people. But healed people can heal people. We take what we learned, good and bad. We help others when we can. Even the smallest gesture can have the most significant impact.

Think for a moment. Do you remember the worst moment of your entire life? Do you remember the situation clearly? Do you remember how you felt when it happened? I bet you do, just like the rest of us.

Now... answer the following question aloud. I don't care where you are or who you're around. Just answer this aloud to yourself... Did you survive? The answer is obviously "Yes." Now, look around you. Even if you're not in an ideal situation right now, appreciate where you are. If you can survive your worst experience, you can survive anything. You're living proof that each and every one of us can keep going.

Our journey together has now come to an end. But this is only the beginning of a new one for you. We may not know each other, but I wish you the best.

ACKNOWLEDGEMENTS

As we reach the end of this book, I want to take a moment to express my gratitude to the people who make this journey called life an extraordinary and meaningful adventure. We are nothing without those who believe in us, support us wholeheartedly, and offer both critiques and encouragement when we need them the most.

I dedicate this book to my incredible family and friends who have challenged me, nurtured me, and laughed alongside me as I turned my dream of "writing a book" into a reality. Your unwavering support means the world to me, and I cannot thank you enough for believing in my vision.

I would not have been able to craft such a cohesive book without the support and guidance of my copy editors, Erin Taylor and Gabrielle Gerbus, who provided key insights and refined my tone and style. I wouldn't have been able to curate such beautiful images and ideas without Yoshino, Allen, Gloria, Kyle, and so many other special friends who helped me create order out of chaos. Thank you to A.J., who was a significant inspiration for creating this book in the first place.

To the kind strangers who have crossed my path and shared their personal stories, you have inspired me, taught me valuable lessons, and fueled my desire to make a positive impact in this world. Your resilience in the face of adversity is a testament to the power of perseverance and serves as a constant reminder that we're never alone in our struggles.

As you reflect on the words and ideas presented in this book, remember to find joy in the journey, draw inspiration from those around you, and always know that we're in this together. Our collective determination is unstoppable, and I'm excited to see where it takes us. From the bottom of my heart, thank you for being a part of my story and for allowing me the privilege of being a part of yours.

NOTES

1   Barker, E. (2015, August 27). How to Increase Mental Toughness: 4 Secrets of Navy SEALs and Olympians. Observer. https://observer.com/2015/08/how-to-increase-mental-toughness-4-secrets-of-navy-seals-and-olympians/#:~:text=Your%20brain%20is%20always%20going,words%20need%20to%20be%20positive

2   Chen, D. (2017, April 12). 4 lessons from the longest-running study on happiness. Ted Talks. https://ideas.ted.com/4-lessons-from-the-longest-running-study-on-happiness/

3   Clifford, C. (2017, January 19). GoPro founder shares how he went from selling shells out of his van to the CEO of a billion-dollar company. CNBC. https://www.cnbc.com/2017/01/09/ceo-of-billion-dollar-company-gopro-shares-his-secret-to-success.html

4   Collins, B. (2014, November 14). 4 Simple Remedies for Burnout backed by science. Fast Company. https://www.fastcompany.com/3038545/4-simple-remedies-for-burnout-backed-by-science

5   Ehrlich, B. (2013, February 14). Why it's really possible to fall in love online. CNN Business. https://www.cnn.com/2013/02/14/tech/social-media/online-love/index.html

6   Elflein, J. (2018, November 21). Common daily life stressors among U.S. Generation Z adults in 2018. Statista. https://www.statista.com/statistics/943836/life-stressors-for-generation-z-adults-us/

7   Ellithorpe ME, Ulusoy E, Eden A, et al. The complicated impact of media use before bed on sleep: Results from a combination of objective EEG sleep measurement and media diaries. J Sleep Res. 2022;31(5):e13551. doi:10.1111/jsr.13551

8   Exelmans L, et al. (2017). Binge viewing, sleep, and the role of pre-sleep arousal. DOI: https://doi.org/10.5664/jcsm.6704

9   Exelmans L, Van den Bulck J. The use of media as a sleep aid in adults. Behav Sleep Med. 2016;14(2):121-133. doi:10.1080/15402002.2014.963582

10   Frankl, V. E. (1959). Man's Search for Meaning. Verlag für Jugend und Volk (Austria) and Beacon Press (English).

11   Hysing M, Pallesen S, Stormark KM, et al. Sleep and use of electronic devices in adolescence: Results from a large population-based study. BMJ Open. 2015;5(1):e006748. doi:10.1136/bmjopen-2014-006748

12   Jardine, R. (2018, August 2). Your Habits Determine Your Chances of Success. Entrepreneur. https://www.entrepreneur.com/en-za/growth-strategies/your-habits-determine-your-chances-of-success/328407

13   Jeffries, S. (2015, October 21). Why too much choice is stressing us. The Guardian. https://www.theguardian.com/lifeandstyle/2015/oct/21/choice-stressing-us-out-dating-partners-monopolies

14   Khullar, D. (2018, January 1). Finding Purpose for a Good Life. But Also a Healthy One. New York Times. https://www.nytimes.com/2018/01/01/upshot/finding-purpose-for-a-good-life-but-also-a-healthy-one.html

15   Kristensen, T., Borritz, M., Villadsen, E., & Christensen, K. (2005). The Copenhagen Burnout Inventory: A new tool for the assessment of burnout. Work and Stress, 19, 192-207. https://doi.org/10.1080/02678370500297720

16   Mac, R. (2016, January 13). Nick Woodman No Longer A Billionaire As GoPro Shares Nosedive. Forbes. https://www.forbes.com/sites/ryanmac/2016/01/13/gopro-nick-woodman-no-longer-a-billionaire/#:~:text=At%20that%20time%2C%20Woodman%20had,beyond%20its%20trademark%20action%20cameras

17 Martini, E. A. (2018). The Placebo Effect: Reflections on Ken Burns's and Lynn Novick's The Vietnam War. Diplomatic History. https://doi.org/10.1093/dh/dhy013

18 Maslach, C., Jackson, S., & Leiter, M. (1997). The Maslach Burnout Inventory Manual. In *Evaluating Stress: A Book of Resources* (Vol. 3, pp. 191-218).

19 Mineo, L. (2017, April 17). Good genes are nice, but joy is better. The Harvard Gazette. https://news.harvard.edu/gazette/story/2017/04/over-nearly-80-years-harvard-study-has-been-showing-how-to-live-a-healthy-and-happy-life/

20 Morin, A. (2015, April 10). 5 Reasons Studies Say You Have to Choose Your Friends Wisely. Psychology Today. https://www.psychologytoday.com/us/blog/what-mentally-strong-people-dont-do/201504/5-reasons-studies-say-you-have-choose-your-friends#:~:text=A%202013%20study%20published%20in,a%20stealth%20secret%20to%20success

21 National Institute on Aging. A good night's sleep.

22 National Institute of Neurological Disorders and Stroke. Brain basics: Understanding sleep.

23 National Sleep Foundation. National Sleep Foundation's Sleep in America poll: Americans can do more during the day to help their sleep at night.

24 National Institutes of Health (NIH). (n.d.). Breaking Bad Habits Why It's So Hard to Change. National Institutes of Health (NIH). https://newsinhealth.nih.gov/2012/01/breaking-bad-habits

25 National Institute of Neurological Disorders and Stroke. Brain basics: Understanding sleep.

26 National Institutes of Health (NIH). (n.d.). Breaking Bad Habits Why It's So Hard to Change. National Institutes of Health (NIH). https://newsinhealth.nih.gov/2012/01/breaking-bad-habits

27 Newport, C. (2016). Deep Work: Rules for Focused Success in a Distracted World. Grand Central Publishing.

28 Novotney, A. (n.d.). The risks of social isolation. New York Times. https://www.apa.org/monitor/2019/05/ce-corner-isolation

29 Ramcharan, Aaron. 2022. "The Social Axiom Framework: Towards a Renaissance of Sustainability." Texas Law Review 100 (7): 1433.

30 Salecl, R. (2011). The Tyranny of Choice (Big Ideas). Profile Books.

31 Savoie, G. (2021, May 9). A Relationship Expert Explains How Social Media Affects Your Love Life. Brides. https://www.brides.com/how-social-media-affects-relationships-5105350

32 Schwartz, B. (2004). The Paradox of Choice: Why More Is Less. Harper Perennial.

33 Shechter A, Kim EW, St-Onge MP, et al. Blocking nocturnal blue light for insomnia: A randomized controlled trial. J Psychiatr Res. 2018;96:196-202. doi:10.1016/j.jpsychires.2017.10.015

34 St.Amant, T. (2017). The Effect of Teacher Mindset on Low-Tracked Students. https://core.ac.uk/download/83547848.pdf

35 Starosta J, et al. (2020). Understanding the phenomenon of binge-watching - A systematic review. DOI: https://doi.org/10.3390/ijerph17124469

36 Thompson, R. (2020, September 18). How To Set Boundaries In The Early Stages Of Dating. Mashable. https://in.mashable.com/culture/17094/how-to-set-boundaries-in-the-early-stages-of-dating

37 Tsuno N, et al. (2005). Sleep and depression. DOI: https://doi.org/10.4088/jcp.v66n1008

38   Vinall, M. (n.d.). Can Horror Movies Negatively Impact Your Mental Health? Healthline. https://www.healthline.com/health/how-do-horror-movies-affect-your-mental-health

39   Walker M. P, et al. (2009). Overnight therapy? The role of sleep in emotional brain processing. DOI: https://doi.org/10.1037/a0016570

40   Waters F, et al. (2018). Severe sleep deprivation causes hallucinations and a gradual progression toward psychosis with increasing time awake. DOI: https://doi.org/10.3389/fpsyt.2018.00303

41   West, H. (2017, December 22). What Causes Fear of Failure and How to Conquer It with Self-Acceptance. Harper West. https://www.harperwest.co/what-causes-fear-of-failure-how-conquer-with-self-acceptance/

42   Yoon H, Baek HJ. External auditory stimulation as a non-pharmacological sleep aid. Sensors (Basel). 2022;22(3):1264. doi:10.3390/s22031264